Neurological Rehabilitation of Multiple Sclerosis

Edited by

Alan J Thompson MD FRCP FRCPI

Head, Rehabilitation Group and Clinical Director
Institute of Neurology, University College London
National Hospital for Neurology and Neurosurgery
London, UK

informa
healthcare

© 2006 Informa UK Ltd

First published in the United Kingdom in 2006 by Informa UK Ltd,
4 Park Square, Milton Park, Abingdon, Oxon OX14 4RN
Informa Healthcare is a trading division of Informa UK Ltd,
Registered Office: 37/41 Mortimer Street, London W1T 3JH.
Registered in England and Wales Number 1072954.

Tel: +44 (0)20 7017 6000
Fax: +44 (0)20 7017 6699
Email: info.medicine@tandf.co.uk
Website: www.informahealthcare.com

A CIP record for this book is available from the British Library.
Library of Congress Cataloging-in-Publication Data

Data available on application

ISBN10 1 84184 559 0
ISBN13 978 1 84184 559 3

Distributed in North and South America by
Taylor & Francis
6000 Broken Sound Parkway, NW, (Suite 300)
Boca Raton, FL 33487, USA

Within Continental USA
Tel: 800 272 7737; Fax: 800 374 3401
Outside Continental USA
Tel: 561 994 0555; Fax: 561 361 6018
Email: orders@crcpress.com

Distributed in the rest of the world by
Thomson Publishing Services
Cheriton House
North Way
Andover, Hampshire SP10 5BE, UK
Tel: +44 (0)1264 332424
Email: tps.tandfsalesorder@thomson.com

Composition by Scribe Design Ltd, Ashford, Kent, UK
Printed and bound in India by Replika Press Pvt Ltd

Neurological Rehabilitation
of Multiple Sclerosis

Queen Square Neurological Rehabilitation Series

Series Editor

Alan J Thompson MD FRCP FRCPI

Head, Rehabilitation Group and Clinical Director
Institute of Neurology, University College London
National Hospital for Neurology & Neurosurgery
London, UK

Contents

Contributors

Stefan J Cano PhD CPsychol
Lecturer
Neurological Outcome
    Measures Unit
Peninsula Medical School
Plymouth
and
Institute of Neurology
London, UK

Olga Ciccarelli PhD
Wellcome Advanced Fellow
Department of Headache, Brain
    Injury and Rehabilitation
Institute of Neurology
and
Honorary Consultant
    Neurologist
National Hospital for Neurology
    and Neurosurgery
London, UK

**Jennifer A Freeman BAppSci
    PhD MCSP**
Honorary Lecturer
Institute of Neurology
London, UK
and
Reader in Physiotherapy and
    Rehabilitation
Faculty of Health and Social
    Work
Plymouth University
Plymouth, UK

Jeremy C Hobart
Senior Lecturer
Neurological Outcome
    Measures Unit
Peninsula Medical School
Plymouth, UK
and
Institute of Neurology
London, UK

Charles Morland
Occasional patient of National
    Hospital for Neurology and
    Neurosurgery
London, UK

Ben Murphy MEng&man, ACA
MS patient of National Hospital
    for Neurology and
    Neurosurgery
London, UK

E Diane Playford MD FRCP
Senior Lecturer and Consultant
National Hospital for Neurology
    and Neurosurgery
London, UK

Bernadette Porter RGN MSc
Nurse Consultant – Multiple
    Sclerosis
National Hospital for Neurology
    and Neurosurgery
London, UK

Valerie L Stevenson MD MRCP
Consultant Neurologist
National Hospital for Neurology
   and Neurosurgery
London, UK

Ahmed T Toosy PhD
Senior Specialist Registrar in
   Neurology
Department of Headache, Brain
   Injury and Rehabilitation
Institute of Neurology
London, UK

Series Preface

Neurological rehabilitation aims to lessen the impact of neurological disorders and minimize their impact on those affected by them. The importance of managing the consequences of acute and chronic neurological disorders is increasingly acknowledged, as is the role that neurologists can and should play. This has required a broader focus for neurological practice, which, in turn, has a major implication for training.

This series, written by people from a variety of backgrounds, is an attempt to deliver the essentials of neurological rehabilitation in a concise and user-friendly fashion. It will cover a range of neurological disorders, all of which have a major impact on those affected. The third in the series aims to provide an evidence base for rehabilitation in multiple sclerosis. It brings together a multidisciplinary team of experts, and it is hoped that by publishing the essential elements in a concise and accessible format it will prove a useful aid in patient management.

Alan J Thompson
Series Editor

Preface

There can be few conditions that test management resources to the extent that occurs in multiple sclerosis (MS). The unpredictable and variable course of this incurable condition, its diverse symptoms and complex disability together represent a major challenge to any health service delivery. In addition, this chronic condition can cause acute and serious disabling symptoms, which require a rapid and effective response. People tend to be affected at a critical time in their lives when they have young families and are building up their careers, thus the impact of this condition goes far beyond those who are diagnosed and affects their family, friends, employers and the society in which they are active members.

Numerous national and international documents and guidelines have shown us that people with MS benefit from comprehensive information on all aspects of their condition and easy access to an expert, multidisciplinary service which is both responsive and co-ordinated. Communication is key!

In this short book we have again focussed on the critical elements inherent to effective rehabilitation – an understanding of the mechanisms underlying disability and recovery in MS, an appreciation of the impact the condition has on those affected by it and the key elements of rehabilitation and service delivery. The authors include neuroscientists, neurologists, psychometricians, MS nurse specialists, therapists and people affected by MS. This reflects the key elements of the multi-disciplinary team which is fundamental to the effective management of this condition. This slim volume is written in a concise and accessible style and will be an easy resource for all of those involved in the rehabilitation of MS.

Alan J Thompson

Mechanisms of disability and potential for recovery in multiple sclerosis

Olga Ciccarelli and Ahmed T Toosy

Introduction

Multiple sclerosis (MS) is an autoimmune central nervous system (CNS) disorder, characterized pathologically by disseminated inflammatory demyelination and neuronal loss. A central concept in understanding relapsing–remitting MS pathophysiology is that of plaque evolution. This is related to pathological processes affecting the complex oligodendrocyte–axon unit.[1] The oligodendrocyte synthesizes and maintains myelin that ensheaths neighboring axons and ensures efficient axonal conduction. In acute inflammatory lesions (plaques) the oligodendrocyte is targeted by immune attack. This is thought to arise from a breakdown in immune self-tolerance, leading to the entry into the CNS of autoreactive T cells across the blood–brain barrier. An inflammatory cycle is then established, comprising mainly activated T cells and microglia. The subsequent release of toxic inflammatory mediators results in axonal and glial injury, and the breakdown of myelin with conduction block (Figure 1.1). These processes manifest with the acute neurological symptoms seen in an MS relapse. In particular, the symptomatology depends upon

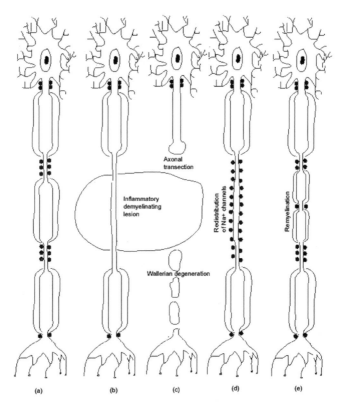

Figure 1.1   Axonal pathology and remyelination in MS. (a) Normal axon. (b) Demyelination within the inflammatory lesion. (c) Axon undergoes Wallerian degeneration distal to the site of transaction. (d) Redistribution of sodium channel and resolution of inflammation contribute to clinical recovery. (e) Remyelination restores conduction and contributes to remission.

the CNS region affected by the acute inflammatory plaque (Figure 1.2). For example, involvement of the optic nerve results in optic neuritis, a very common disorder in MS which results in visual loss.

Repair mechanisms, that include resolution of inflammation, restoration of conduction in demyelinated axons, remyelination

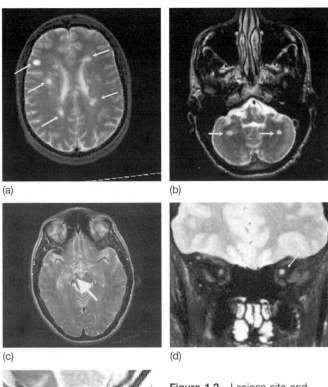

(a) (b)

(c) (d)

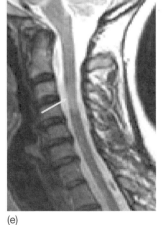

(e)

Figure 1.2 Lesions site and symptoms

MS lesions appear as areas of high signal intensity on axial T2 weighted images (arrows). (a) Cerebrum; (b) cerebellum; (c) right cerebral peduncle in the brainstem; (d) left optic nerve (coronal PD fat-saturated FSE image); (e) cervical spinal cord (longitudinal section)

continued overleaf

Lesion site	Cerebrum	Cerebellum	Brainstem	Optic nerve	Spinal cord
Symptoms	Cognitive impairment Hemisensory and motor Affective (mainly depression) Focal cortical deficits (rare) Epilepsy (rare)	Tremor Lack of limb coordination Poor balance Clumsiness Speech problems	Visual disturbances Vertigo Impaired speech and swallowing Paroxysmal symptoms	Unilateral painful loss of vision Visual field defects	Lhermitte Limb weakness Stiffness and painful spasms Bladder dysfunction Erectile impotence Constipation

(The above table is adapted from reference 1)

(Figure 1.1) and, perhaps, cortical adaptation, spontaneously occur within the lesions, and are responsible for the clinical recovery phase of a relapse.

Commonly, early MS is distinguished by frequent relapses, suggesting significant inflammatory activity during this part of the illness. Over time, as the condition enters a progressive phase, the relapse frequency abates. This phase is dominated pathologically by neuronal loss that is thought to be of multifactorial etiology. Permanent axonal loss resulting from incomplete reparative processes may contribute, for example, to persistent clinical deficit.[2] Other contributing factors include Wallerian degeneration following transection of axons in the inflammatory lesions, and astrocyte reactivity resulting in gliosis, further impeding any regenerative capacity.[1] In addition there is accumulating evidence for neuronal loss that cannot be explained by the consequences of acute inflammatory macroscopic lesions. Magnetic resonance imaging (MRI) and post-mortem evidence implicates disease involvement of normal appearing white matter (NAWM) and normal appearing gray matter (NAGM) that may contribute to progressive brain atrophy (Figure 1.3), a sensitive marker for the neurodegenerative aspect of MS. This is now felt to commence early on in the condition.[3,4]

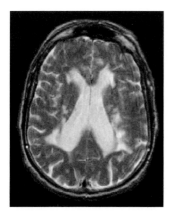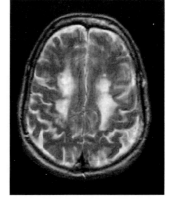

Figure 1.3 Atrophy in MS appears as increased size of the ventricles and cortical sulci on MRI images

Interesting work has also revealed a more complicated patho-logical scenario than was previously realized. A pathological study classified actively demyelinating plaques from MS patients into four categories of tissue injury:[5] (1) T cell/macrophage-associated demyelination; (2) antibody/complement-associated demyelination; (3) oligodendrocyte dystrophy with myelin protein dysregulation and oligodendrocyte apoptosis; (4) primary oligo-dendrocyte degeneration with features similar to those of viral infection or toxic oligodendrocyte damage, but not to those of autoimmunity. It was suggested that individual MS patients would possess only one of these four pathological subtypes, although these patterns were distributed homogeneously among the differ-ent disease courses. Another study has questioned our under-standing of the pathology in relapsing–remitting MS by showing extensive oligodendrocyte apoptosis and microglial activation in myelinated tissue containing few or no lymphocytes or myelin phagocytes in 12 patients.[6] These studies may have implications for our understanding of disease progression and its potential treatment.

In this chapter we review the pathophysiology of the disease, and link the pathological processes to the clinical features of MS. We will often refer to optic neuritis because it is an excellent model to study the mechanisms of damage and repair in the CNS, through the ability of MRI to visualise the optic nerves, and of visual evoked potentials (VEPs) to assess the optic nerve conduc-tion. Furthermore, the visual symptoms caused by an episode of optic neuritis usually resolve. The pathophysiological mecha-nisms may be divided into those that account for negative symptoms or loss of function, recovery of function and positive phenomena. At the end of this chapter we will discuss the mechanisms of persistent neurological deficit.

Negative symptoms

Effects of demyelination

Negative symptoms are primarily due to the loss of conduction within a nerve. A major cause is axonal conduction block, in which the transmission of electrical impulse trains along the axon is interrupted, and this has been reliably localized to the sites of demyelination (Figure 1.1).[7,8] Under experimental conditions, following segmental demyelination of the sciatic nerve, spinal roots or dorsal columns, conduction block tends to persist for the first few days[9] and this is thought to be related to an initial paucity of sodium channels in the underlying axolemma.[10] Widening of the nodal gap may also cause conduction block and this is thought to arise from a reduction in the safety factor[a] for conduction.[11] This reduction is due to an increase in nodal membrane area, which will raise the electrical capacitance and will also dissipate the local depolarizing nodal currents.[12]

Effects of inflammation

Inflammation has also been implicated in contributing to conduction block. A strong relationship was demonstrated between contrast enhancement on MRI of the optic nerve and reduced VEP amplitude during the acute phase when vision was poor.[13] One month later, after visual recovery, the VEP amplitude had returned towards normal, indicating partial recovery of conduction block. In addition, contrast enhancement on MRI was no longer evident; however, VEP delay was still present, consistent with persistent demyelination. This suggested that the onset and resolution of inflammation contributes to the onset and recovery of conduction block (and clinical deficit).

Pro-inflammatory cytokines probably mediate the mechanisms that contribute to conduction block. The cytokines tumor necrosis factor-α (TNF-α) and interferon-γ (IFN-γ) have been implicated, and although direct effects on axonal conduction have been difficult to detect,[14] they are known to promote the expression of the inducible form of nitric oxide synthase (iNOS).[15,16] Evidence for the putative role of nitric oxide (NO) in mediating the inflammatory process is strengthened by the finding that its synthesis is raised in MS and in inflammatory lesions.[17,18] In addition, physiological levels of NO have been shown to cause conduction block in both normal[19,20] and demyelinated axons.[19] Potential therapies could attempt to reduce NO levels in the future. For example, the animal model of experimental autoimmune encephalomyelitis has demonstrated the benefit of using

---

[a]The safety factor for conduction is the ratio of the actual local action current that depolarizes a node to the minimum current that is necessary to do so. It is around three to five in normal axons but in demyelinated axons it is near unity, making conduction less reliable.

NOX-100, an NO scavenger, which greatly reduces disease progression in combination with the immunosuppressant cyclosporin A in mice.[21]

Inflammation may also alter glial cell properties, in particular those of astrocytes and microglia, which could contribute to neurological dysfunction.[22,23] Astrocytes are thought to regulate chemical factors in the brain and are physically associated with neurons, dendrites, synapses and nodes of Ranvier.[24]

Recovery of function

Conduction recovery in demyelinated axons

Studies of experimentally demyelinated central axons have shown that conduction tends to recover within 2–3 weeks of demyelination.[25] It is believed that this recovery is helped by the appearance of sodium channels along the demyelinated axolemma[26] (Figure 1.1) and also by the restored conduction being more continuous, as is the case with peripheral demyelinated axons,[27] rather than saltatory. A recent study found these sodium channels to belong to the Na 1.6 and Na 1.2 isoforms in acute MS lesions from the cervical cord and optic nerve.[28]

Resolution of inflammation

Clinical recovery following optic neuritis is associated with a concomitant reduction of contrast enhancement on optic nerve MRI, which suggests that it may be influenced by the resolution of inflammation.[13] Further supportive evidence is provided by the observation that NO-induced conduction block is reversed when the agent is removed.[19]

Role of remyelination

Remyelination is common in MS[29,30] and is effective at restoring conduction;[31,32] however, the newly myelinated internodes are shorter and thinner than normal (Figure 1.1). Despite this, the conduction efficacy is thought to be reasonably well maintained at physiological frequencies.[33]

Although remyelination is known to start within a few days of the inflammatory lesion onset, there is evidence that remyelination may continue for more than 2 years. A paper reported the findings of one cross-sectional and two longitudinal studies[34] and described how the VEP latencies continued to shorten over the next 2–3 years despite negligible improvements in visual recovery. The long-term VEP latency evolution was attributed to myelin repair processes that may protect the demyelinated axons from subsequent degeneration. The authors also noted an asymptomatic deterioration in the VEPs of the fellow eyes, possibly due to latent demyelination or axonal degeneration.

Role of cortical adaptation

Certain aspects of functional recovery cannot be explained by structural mechanisms such as the resolution of inflammation or edema. Alterations in distributed cortical processing related to certain clinical functions may occur. This cortical plasticity has been postulated to contribute to clinical recovery.

The term cortical plasticity has been defined as the 'reorganisation of distributed patterns of normal task-associated brain activity that accompany action, perception, and cognition and that compensate impaired function resulting from disease or brain injury.'[35] Although the capacity for cortical plasticity is at its greatest during the early years of CNS development, it appears to persist throughout life. The behavioral effects of cortical reorganization following CNS insult may be divided into different categories which describe, for example, adaptive and maladaptive processes. Adaptive cortical reorganization implies that the redistribution of neural processing in some way contributes to the mechanisms involved in clinical recovery or helps to maintain a degree of clinical function in the presence of structural damage. At least four forms of adaptive plasticity have been suggested.[36] (1) Homologous area adaptation – implies that the damaged brain region can be compensated for by transferring the neural operations to other unaffected brain modules (usually in the homologous region of the opposite hemisphere). (2) Cross-modal reassignment – occurs when cortical modules usually devoted to processing particular sensory inputs now accept inputs from another sensory modality. (3) Map expansion – is the enlargement of a functional cortical region in response to frequent stimulus exposure or following adjacent cortical injury. (4) Compensatory masquerade – is the novel allocation of a cognitive strategy to perform a task that otherwise would depend on another cognitive process which is now impaired.

Table 1.1. Summary of some selected fMRI studies in MS

Author and date	Patients studied	Paradigm	Main findings	Conclusions
Werring, 2000[43]	CIS (ON)	Visual	Reduced activation in visual cortex and greater activation in extra-occipital areas (ex. insula)	Activation of areas outside visual cortex contribute to recovery
Toosy, 2005[46]	CIS (ON)	Visual	Reduced activation in visual cortex and activation of lateral occipital complexes (high order areas)	Adaptive role for cortical reorganization within lateral occipital complexes
Rocca, 2003[47]	CIS	Upper limb – motor	Increased activation in contr. sensorimotor cortex that correlates with reduced NAA	Adaptive cortical plasticity within the contr. sensorimotor cortex
Pantano, 2002[48]	CIS (hemi-paresis and ON)	Upper limb – motor	Greater activation in ips. sensorimotor cortex, parietal cortex and insula, and in contr. motor cortex. Correlations between fMRI and T2 and T1 lesion loads in the corticospinal tracts	Contribution of corticospinal tract damage to cortical motor reorganization after hemiparesis
Rocca, 2003[50]	CIS (myelitis)	Upper limb – motor	Greater activation in ips. primary sensorimotor cortex, suppl. motor area and middle frontal gyrus that correlates with spinal cord MTR	Adaptive cortical plasticity within the middle frontal gyrus after cord damage
Reddy, 2000[53]	RR MS	Upper limb – motor	Greater activation at 3 and 6 weeks in contr. and ips. motor areas. Normal activation at 6 months	Dynamic fMRI changes following acute subcortical injury
Lee, 2000[52]	RR MS	Upper limb – motor	Greater activation in ips. suppl. motor cortex that correlates with lesion load	Cortical reorganization or 'unmasking' of latent pathways contribute to recovery
Reddy, 2000[51]	RR MS	Upper limb – motor	Greater activation in ips. sensorimotor cortex and central white matter NAA	Adaptive cortical reorganization compensates for axonal injury in the corticospinal tract

Study	Group	Task	Results	Conclusions
Reddy, 2002[54]	RR and RP MS	Upper limb – motor	Differences in activation between subgroups with different hand function or brain injury	Disability and structural brain injury contribute to changes in the fMRI patterns
Staffen, 2002[56]	RR MS	Cognitive task – Paced Visual Serial Addition	Greater activation in frontal and parietal areas	Compensatory cortical plasticity within frontal and parietal regions, as a result of raised cerebral effort
Mainero, 2004[55]	RR MS	Cognitive task – PASAT and recall test	Greater activation in several areas (suppl. motor area, cingulate, prefrontal, temporal and parietal areas, and basal ganglia)	Brain reorganization during attention, information processing and memory tasks
Rocca, 2003[50]	SP MS	Upper and lower limb – motor	Greater activation in areas within the motor network that correlate with NAWM and NAGM damage	Cortical plasticity within highly specialized cortical areas limits the impact of MS-related damage
Rocca, 2002[59]	PP MS	Upper and lower limb – motor	Greater activation in a widespread cortical pattern	Cortical plasticity involves regions associated with multimodal integration
Filippi, 2002[60]	PP MS	Upper limb – motor	Correlations between activation in sensorimotor areas and several measures of brain and cord structural pathology	Compensatory mechanisms preserve clinical function in response to structural damage
Ciccarelli, 2006[61]	PP MS	Lower limb – motor	Greater activation with passive movements in regions that participate in sensorimotor integration (ex. putamen). Activation in ips. inferior frontal gyrus and contr. cerebellum was lower in patients with greater disability	Increased activation with passive movements reflects true functional reorganization. There is a loss of distributed activation in more disabled patients

CIS, clinically isolated syndrome; ON, optic neuritis; contr., contralateral; ips., ipsilateral; suppl., supplementary; RR, relapsing–remitting; PP, primary progressive; SP, secondary progressive; NAA, N-acetylaspartate; MTR, magnetization transfer ratio

However, cortical reorganization may not necessarily contribute to recovery of clinical function. It may also reflect the recruitment of unusual distributed neural networks purely as a 'stress' response to CNS injury, implying that it can be non-adaptive. Indeed, plastic changes, in response to injury, may also have deleterious behavioral effects resulting in functional loss rather than gain. This form of plasticity is termed 'maladaptive' and is, for example, thought to account for phantom limb pain following amputation.[37]

Functional neuroimaging has demonstrated cortical plasticity in demyelinating disease. Studies have employed functional MRI (fMRI) with experimental paradigms for the visual and the motor systems and have addressed clinically isolated syndromes such as optic neuritis, relapsing–remitting MS, secondary progressive MS and primary progressive MS.

There are some interpretational caveats that may limit the inferences about the functional nature of cortical reorganization after neurological insult. First, there is an implicit assumption, when comparing patients with neurological disease with healthy controls, that the neurovascular coupling mechanisms generating the BOLD response are similar. This may not be the case; for example, it is possible that vasoactive substances derived from inflammatory lesions could alter the spatiotemporal dynamics of the BOLD response. In practice, it tends not to be considered important and may be more relevant with event-related fMRI studies.

Second, with motor tasks, there should be careful control of task performance between individuals, as it is well known that task complexity[38,39] and effort[40] will affect the resulting brain activation patterns. A related issue concerns the decision to control for absolute or relative biomechanical parameters (e.g. with movement frequency and amplitude or force generation). Although the studies described in the following sections and summarized in Table 1.1 tended to control for absolute mechanical parameters (in particular movement frequency), some experimenters control for individual relative effort. They reason that patients, with impaired motor performance, who are asked to perform a motor task with the same absolute parameters as controls will find the task more effortful or cognitively complex, resulting in differences in activation secondary to differences in relative effort. This argument has greater applicability in patients with impaired function.

Third, correlations between fMRI activation and markers of brain damage can be presumed to be adaptive, but could still be non-adaptive. They may constitute a 'stress' or hyperexcitable response of certain cortical regions to diffuse brain injury. It may therefore be difficult to disentangle genuine adaptive cortical plasticity from non-adaptive cortical plasticity.

Clinically isolated syndromes

Previous visual fMRI studies have been mainly cross-sectional and have studied patients with previous optic neuritis (ON).[41–44] The main findings have been reduced fMRI visual cortex activation with occasional evidence for correlations between fMRI activity and visual function or VEP data. Werring et al.[43] demonstrated an extensive extra-occipital pattern of activation in seven ON patients. These extra-occipital regions are known to have connections with primary visual areas in animal models and some are thought to be involved in multimodal sensory integration. A multimodal MRI longitudinal study examined 20 patients with acute ON over 1 year and found that activation differences between patients and controls within the same extra-occipital areas were especially prominent early on after onset.[45] Further analysis of these data correlated the fMRI response to clinical function and optic nerve structural damage in a novel technique that was able to determine the contribution fMRI made to clinical function after accounting for structural factors.[46] Significant effects were found at baseline in the lateral occipital complexes, normally involved in higher-order visual processing, suggesting a genuine adaptive role for cortical reorganization within these areas after ON.

Motor fMRI studies have also been applied to clinically isolated syndromes.[47,48] One study conducted proton magnetic resonance spectroscopy as well as upper limb motor fMRI sequences.[47] Patients, recruited within 3 months of symptom onset, had greater activation of the contralateral sensorimotor cortex, secondary somatosensory cortex and inferior frontal gyrus compared with controls. They also had reduced whole brain N-acetylaspartate (NAA) concentrations (indicating axonal injury) which were inversely correlated with the contralateral sensorimotor cortex fMRI response. As the task performance was matched between patients and controls, it was suggested that the correlation may reflect adaptive cortical plasticity to maintain normal clinical function in the presence of brain neuronal injury.

Another motor fMRI study compared three groups of patients using upper limb motor fMRI – 10 patients with previous hemiparesis, 10 patients with previous ON and 10 controls.[49] The hemiparetic patients demonstrated greater ipsilateral activation within the sensorimotor cortex, parietal cortex and insula and greater contralateral activation in the motor cortex. There was also a positive correlation between markers of damage for the corticospinal tracts (T2 and T1 lesion loads) and activation of several motor-related areas from both hemispheres, suggesting that the corticospinal tract damage contributes to cortical motor reorganization after hemiparesis.

Single-episode spinal cord relapses (myelitis) have also been investigated using fMRI. A study investigated 14 patients with previous cervical myelitis and normal upper limb function.[50] Upper limb motor fMRI and diffusion tensor imaging (DTI) of the brain were conducted as well as magnetization transfer imaging and conventional MRI of the cervical cord and brain. Compared with healthy volunteers, the myelitis patients had significantly greater activations in the ipsilateral primary sensorimotor cortex, supplementary motor area and middle frontal gyrus. The average cervical cord magnetization transfer ratio was inversely correlated with activations within the middle frontal and ipsilateral postcentral gyri, suggesting a possible role for adaptive cortical plasticity.

Relapsing–remitting multiple sclerosis

Several motor fMRI studies have investigated cortical reorganization in MS. An early study serially scanned a relapsing–remitting MS patient during the recovery period of a right hemiplegic relapse, which was associated with a left hemisphere demyelinating lesion.[51] Magnetic resonance spectroscopy and fMRI were performed over 6 months following presentation. The NAA concentration in the affected corticospinal tract increased in parallel with clinical recovery. The fMRI activation was larger at 3 and 6 weeks, compared with controls, in contra- and ipsilateral motor areas, whereas at 6 months it had returned to control levels. Clinical function had recovered by 6 weeks and remained stable thereafter. This study demonstrated dynamic changes in the motor fMRI response following acute subcortical injury even after the completion of clinical recovery.

In a follow-up study by Lee et al., greater ipsilateral motor cortex activation was demonstrated in a group of 12 MS patients compared with 12 healthy controls.[52] A lateralization index was calculated to quantify the contralateral bias and was found to inversely correlate with disease burden as measured by the T2 lesion load. In particular, greater ipsilateral supplementary motor cortex activation extent positively correlated with lesion load. A posterior shift in the activation center by 8.8 mm of the contralateral supplementary motor cortex in patients relative to controls was also reported. The authors surmised that these results could reflect adaptive cortical plasticity.

Some studies have used MS patients with normal upper limb function in an attempt to avoid confounding influences of differences between patient and control performance. Reddy et al. compared nine MS patients who had unimpaired upper limb hand function with eight normal controls.[53] The authors demonstrated a fivefold increase in sensorimotor cortex activation for the MS patients relative to normal controls. They also reported a significant correlation between the volume of ipsilateral sensorimotor cortex activation and the central white matter NAA. It was felt that, although the corticospinal tracts were not selectively sampled, the central white matter NAA measurements still reflected corticospinal tract pathology. The authors suggested that adaptive cortical reorganization had occurred to compensate for axonal injury presumably to the corticospinal tracts in order to maintain hand function.

Clinical disability itself is known to be associated with altered patterns of cortical activation. This relationship may simply reflect the expected dependence of disability on structural brain injury but it may also be directly related to disability, such as altered patterns of use. An upper limb motor fMRI study was designed to investigate this by selecting three groups of patients with relapsing–remitting or relapsing–progressive MS:[54] (1) group 1 – normal hand function and low levels of white matter injury; (2) group 2 – normal hand function and higher levels of white matter injury; (3) group 3 – reduced hand function and higher levels of white matter injury. Contrasts between groups 2 and 1 showed greater activation within the supplementary motor area bilaterally and premotor cortex ipsilaterally for group 2. A comparison between groups 2 and 3 revealed greater primary and secondary somatosensory, as well as parietal cortex activation, in group 3. This was interpreted as a disability-related reorganization of brain function and the authors felt therefore that both clinical disability and structural brain injury may contribute to changes in the patterns of movement-associated brain activation.

In addition to motor fMRI, cognitive tasks have been investigated using fMRI in MS. Staffen et al. found greater activation for frontal and parietal areas in relapsing–remitting MS patients with mild disability[55] compared with controls during the Paced Visual Serial Addition Task. They felt that this represented compensatory cortical plasticity for the MS patients, possibly as a result of raised cerebral effort. Another study investigated the fMRI activation in 22 patients with no or only mild deficits at neuropsychological testing and 22 healthy subjects during the Paced Auditory Serial Addition Test (PASAT) and a recall task.[56] During both tasks, patients exhibited significantly greater activation and recruited additional brain areas, suggesting that brain reorganization occurs during tasks exploring sustained attention, information processing and memory. Task-related functional changes were more significant in patients with better cognitive function than in those with lower cognitive function.

Secondary progressive multiple sclerosis

Rocca et al. recently published a study looking at both right upper and right lower limb motor fMRI tasks in 13 patients with secondary progressive MS.[57] They selected patients with clinically unaffected right limbs to avoid task performance confounds. DTI was also performed and showed reduced gray and white matter measures of fractional anisotropy (FA) and diffusivity in patients compared with 15 healthy volunteers. With the upper limb task (finger extension-flexion), compared with controls, the MS patients demonstrated greater activation in the ipsilateral inferior frontal gyrus, middle frontal gyrus, bilaterally and contralateral intraparietal sulcus. For the lower limb task (ankle flexion-extension) the MS patients showed more activation of the contralateral sensorimotor cortex and thalamus and of the ipsilateral sylvian fissure. Some strong correlations were found between the several DTI measures and both motor tasks in the frontal lobes.

Primary progressive multiple sclerosis

Primary progressive MS is characterized by the accumulation of progressive clinical deficit. Affected patients tend to have lower MRI lesion loads although several structural measures of normal appearing brain tissue have pointed towards a more prominent role for axonal degeneration.[58]

FMRI studies with primary progressive MS patients have involved motor paradigms. One study investigated the fMRI response to simple and complex motor tasks in 30 primary progressive patients.[59] The functional response of clinically unaffected limbs was compared with that from 15 healthy volunteers. In the MS group, the simple motor task activated more in the contralateral supplementary motor area, the secondary somatosensory cortex and other frontal and temporal regions, including the insula and superior temporal gyrus. This widespread cortical pattern involved some regions thought to be associated with multimodal integration.

A further study applied fMRI, DTI magnetization transfer and cord imaging in primary progressive MS patients with normal right upper limb function.[60] It reported correlations between the extent of fMRI activation in sensorimotor areas and several measures of brain and cord structural pathology, suggesting the existence of attempted compensatory mechanisms within the brain to preserve clinical function in response to structural damage.

A recent study has investigated functional changes that are associated with active and passive ankle movements in patients with primary progressive MS, in order to assess whether functional reorganization diminishes in more disabled patients. [61] Patients showed greater fMRI activation than controls with passive movements in regions that participate in sensorimotor integration, such as the putamen, suggesting true functional reorganization, since passive movements induce brain activation through sensory afferents only. The fMRI response to active and passive movements in the ipsilateral inferior frontal gyrus was lower in patients with greater disability and greater brain T2 lesion load, respectively (Figure 1.4). Furthermore, the fMRI activation with active movements in the contralateral cerebellum was lower in patients with worse mobility (Figure 1.4). These findings suggest that there is a loss of distributed activation in more disabled patients.

Although many fMRI studies have purported to show adaptive cortical plasticity, in reality it is likely that functional reorganization following neurological injury may comprise a mixture of both adaptive and non-adaptive components. These will be complex, dynamic and dependent upon complex interrelationships both within the reorganized networks and between other neurological subsystems with their cortical substrates and will also be influenced by the structural integrity of the specifically involved neural pathways.

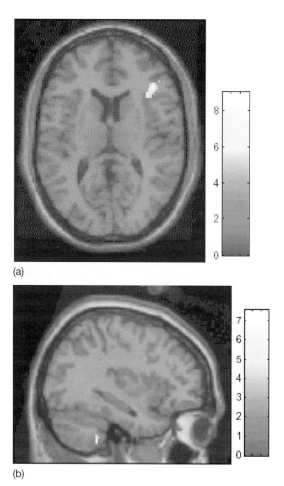

(a)

(b)

Figure 1.4   Results of the correlations between the fMRI response to right ankle movements and clinical scores in patients with primary progressive MS. (a) Activation in the right inferior frontal gyrus (MNI coordinates $x = 42$, $y = 30$, $z = 12$) was lower in patients with higher EDSS. (b) Activation in the left cerebellum ($x = -34$, $y = -42$, $z = -46$) was lower in patients with worse mobility measured by the 25-foot Timed Walked Test. These findings suggest that there is a loss of distributed activation in more disabled patients. Regions of activation are overlaid onto T1-weighted template and corrected for multiple comparisons. The scale indicates the T score

Conduction characteristics following recovery

Conduction slowing

Although recovery of conduction is common following demyelination, the restored conduction itself is neither as fast nor as robust as normal. The low conduction velocity is restricted to the demyelinated portions of the axon and affects the conduction latency.[8] This, along with a reduction in the number of conducting axons, produces latency and waveform changes with VEP testing[62] following acute optic neuritis.

Conduction refractory period of transmission (RPT)

Restored conduction also remains susceptible to conduction block due to a prolonged RPT.[8] This is the maximum interval between two supramaximal stimuli for which the second action potential fails to propagate through the lesion. Repetitively firing impulse trains are attenuated when propagated through the demyelinated lesion, which therefore acts as a reducing frequency filter. This phenomenon may account for the blurring or 'fading' of vision sometimes described with fixated gaze.[63]

Temperature effects

Temperature-sensitive symptomatology is well known following demyelination (Uhthoff's phenomenon). Deleterious changes in visual symptoms occur with warming[64] and conversely improvements in vision with cooling (e.g. cold drinks) are well described.[65] The neurophysiological basis for the beneficial effects of cooling is thought to derive from a small prolongation in action potential duration,[66] itself a consequence of the temperature coefficient for sodium channel inactivation being larger than that for sodium channel activation.[67] In the node prior to the demyelinated region, prolonged action current potentials will encourage depolarization of the demyelinated axon and so enhance nerve conduction.

Positive symptoms

Demyelinated axons can become hyperexcitable and spontaneously generate impulse trains at the site of demyelination which propagate in both directions in experimental models.[68,69]

Several mechanisms have been described which may account for this hyperexcitability. A slow inward sodium current can appear at the sites of demyelination[70,71] and a prolonged, inward potassium current resulting from an accumulation of potassium ions outside the axons has also been reported.[72] In optic neuritis, patients may experience the perception of flashes of light or other phosphenes upon eye movements,[73] which are thought to result from mechanosensitive hyperexcitable properties of demyelinated axons. These axonal properties are also thought to mediate Lhermitte's phenomenon: sensory symptoms, especially 'electric shock'-like sensations, that radiate down the limbs in MS patients on neck flexion.

Ephaptic transmission (cross-talk) can arise between neighboring demyelinated axons, resulting in paroxysmal symptoms, such as trigeminal neuralgia, ataxia, dysarthria, or painful titanic posturing of the limbs, lasting 1 or 2 minutes and often triggered by touch or movement.[1]

Mechanisms of persistent and worsening deficit

Axonal loss

The pathology of axons has been shown to be a major factor in the development of clinical disability. As mentioned above, axonal damage can occur in active lesions,[74,75] due to inflammatory substances that are produced by activated immune and glial cells, and in the NAWM, due to the degeneration of axons transected in focal lesions (Figure 1.1). These transected axons undergo Wallerian degeneration during the subsequent 18 months but this action does not seem to extend the lesion or shape the clinical deficit.[1] The mechanisms that influence the extent of axonal loss are not fully understood, but the severity of early inflammation[76] and also continuing inflammatory processes[77] are thought to be important factors.

Moreover, axonal loss may also occur independently of demyelination, perhaps due to antibodies, anti-axonal proteins, such as the anti-ganglioside antibodies,[78] or to the synthesis of nitric oxide,[79] which can directly damage neurons and axons. A further form of degeneration of axons may occur in those that are chronically demyelinated due to the lack of trophic support from myelin or myelin-forming cells.[80] Therefore, chronic axonal degeneration might slowly increase the clinical deficit, decaying a compromised but functioning pathway and leading to disease progression.

Recent studies in the spinal cord and lateral geniculate body in MS have demonstrated that smaller axons might be more susceptible to damage, and, in particular, to inflammatory mediators, such as nitric oxide (NO), than larger axons.[81]

Clinically, the later stages of MS are characterized by progressive disability and several lines of evidence support the view that axonal loss is probably a major determinant for this. For example, a strong correlation exists between spinal cord atrophy and clinical disability.[82] Various MRI modalities have made important contributions towards determining the mechanisms of atrophy in MS. The interested reader is referred to several comprehensive reviews which cover this topic.[3,4,83,84] Another imaging technique, magnetic resonance spectroscopy, has shown reduced NAA (which is a marker of neuronal dysfunction or loss) in MS lesions and normal-appearing white matter.[85–87] Correlations between NAA, clinical function and cerebellar volumes in MS patients have also been shown.[88] Recent evidence suggests that cerebral atrophy may occur early following a clinically isolated syndrome. In a group of 55 patients with clinically isolated syndromes, ventricular enlargement occurred in the 18 patients who developed clinical MS, and in the 40 patients with abnormal brain MRI at presentation over 1 year. No change in ventricular volume was noted in the 15 patients with normal imaging.[89] Atrophy has also been found early in the disease course of relapsing–remitting MS.[90]

In optic neuritis, there is also evidence for optic atrophy which can continue 3 years after the inflammatory episode. In a serial MRI study, the optic nerve cross-sectional areas were measured in patients 20 months after optic neuritis and one year later.[91] The mean area of the affected optic nerve decreased over 1 year from 11.1 to 10.2 mm^2 (p <0.01). Poor visual acuity and reduced VEP amplitude were associated with optic atrophy. The recently introduced non-invasive technique, optical coherence tomography, has been used to quantify axonal loss of the retinal nerve fiber layer (RNFL) after optic neuritis.[92] RNFL thickness was significantly reduced in the affected patients' eyes compared with healthy volunteers' and clinically unaffected eyes. There were also significant relationships among RNFL thickness and visual acuity, visual field, color vision and VEP amplitude. In addition, a putative role for NO has been suggested in axon degeneration following acute inflammation. Acute Wallerian degeneration has been found in axons of the rat dorsal root ganglion, electrically stimulated at physiological frequencies whilst exposed to low concentrations of NO.[93] Furthermore, a recent study discovered higher plasma biomarkers of axonal injury and higher NO metabolites in patients with acute optic neuritis when compared with healthy volunteers.[94]

Persistent conduction block

This is known to occur in chronic demyelinating peripheral neuropathy[95] and is likely to occur in central demyelinating disease. For instance, if the safety factor in demyelinated axons is around unity, in some axons it will be below unity and this will impose a conduction block that may manifest as persistent clinical deficit.

Conclusions: potential for future treatments

The pathophysiological mechanisms that underpin MS have been shown to be complex, and many issues are still unresolved. However, our understanding of the condition continues to improve and this will help to focus therapeutic strategies on specific components of the inflammatory cascade and/or on the promotion of remyelination and neuroprotection. For example, as the dynamics of spontaneous endogenous demyelination have become clearer, the efforts of the researchers have been aimed to promote remyelination, which may be essential for those demyelinated axons that survive to the inflammation, but could degenerate later due to the lack of trophic support.[80] Enhanced remyelination could be obtained by performing exogenous cell transplantation, and several strategies have been developed in the past few years. Although most of these approaches have been able to form new myelin sheath around the transplantation site, they are very challenging and almost impractical, due to the multifocality and multiphasic course of MS. Recently, promising cell-replacement therapies based on the use of somatic stem cells have been successful in animal studies.[96] However, although somatic stem cells may integrate within the CNS and possibly repair the myelin damage, further studies are needed to assess the efficacy and safety of this approach and solve some of the current issues, such as (1) the ideal stem cell source for transplantation; (2) the route of cell administration; and (3) the long-lasting integration of the transplanted cells into the host tissue.[97]

References

1. Compston A, Coles A (2002) Multiple sclerosis. Lancet 359: 1221–31.

2. Trapp BD, Peterson J, Ransohoff RM et al. (1998) Axonal transection in the lesions of multiple sclerosis. N Engl J Med 338: 278–85.

3. Miller DH, Barkhof F, Frank JA et al. (2002) Measurement of atrophy in multiple sclerosis: pathological basis, methodological aspects and clinical relevance. Brain 125: 1676–95.

4. Miller DH (2004) Biomarkers and surrogate outcomes in neurodegenerative disease: lessons from multiple sclerosis. NeuroRx 1: 284–94.

5. Lucchinetti C, Bruck W, Parisi J et al. (2000) Heterogeneity of multiple sclerosis lesions: implications for the pathogenesis of demyelination. Ann Neurol 47: 707–17.

6. Barnett MH, Prineas JW (2004) Relapsing and remitting multiple sclerosis: pathology of the newly forming lesion. Ann Neurol 55: 458–68.

7. McDonald WI, Sears TA (1969) Effect of demyelination on conduction in the central nervous system. Nature 221: 182–3.

8. McDonald WI, Sears TA (1970) The effects of experimental demyelination on conduction in the central nervous system. Brain 93: 583–98.

9. Smith KJ, McDonald WI (1999) The pathophysiology of multiple sclerosis: the mechanisms underlying the production of symptoms and the natural history of the disease. Philos Trans R Soc Lond B Biol Sci 354: 1649–73.

10. Waxman SG, Ritchie JM (1993) Molecular dissection of the myelinated axon. Ann Neurol 33: 121–36.

11. Tasaki I (1953) Nervous Transmission. Charles C Thomas, Springfield.

12. Smith KJ (1994) Conduction properties of central demyelinated and remyelinated axons, and their relation to symptom production in demyelinating disorders. Eye 8: 224–37.

13. Youl BD, Turano G, Miller DH et al. (1991) The pathophysiology of acute optic neuritis. An association of gadolinium leakage with clinical and electrophysiological deficits. Brain 114: 2437–50.

14. Dugandzija-Novakovic S, Shrager P (1995) Survival, development, and electrical activity of central nervous system myelinated axons exposed to tumor necrosis factor in vitro. J Neurosci Res 40: 117–26.

15. Hu S, Sheng WS, Peterson PK et al. (1995) Differential regulation by cytokines of human astrocyte nitric oxide production. Glia 15: 491–4.

16. Goureau O, Amiot F, Dautry F et al. (1997) Control of nitric oxide production by endogenous TNF-alpha in mouse retinal pigmented epithelial and Muller glial cells. Biochem Biophys Res Commun 240: 132–5.

17. Bo L, Dawson TM, Wesselingh S et al. (1994) Induction of nitric oxide synthase in demyelinating regions of multiple sclerosis brains. Ann Neurol 36: 778–86.

18. Giovannoni G, Heales SJ, Silver NC et al. (1997) Raised serum nitrate and nitrite levels in patients with multiple sclerosis. J Neurol Sci 145: 77–81.

19. Redford EJ, Kapoor R, Smith KJ (1997) Nitric oxide donors reversibly block axonal conduction: demyelinated axons are especially susceptible. Brain 120: 2149–57.

20. Shrager P, Custer AW, Kazarinova K et al. (1998) Nerve conduction block by nitric oxide that is mediated by the axonal environment. J Neurophysiol 79: 529–36.

21. Jolivalt CG, Howard RB, Chen LS et al. (2003) A novel nitric oxide scavenger in combination with cyclosporine A ameliorates experimental autoimmune encephalomyelitis progression in mice. J Neuroimmunol 138: 56–64.

22. Chao CC, Hu S, Peterson PK (1995) Glia, cytokines, and neurotoxicity. Crit Rev Neurobiol 9: 189–205.

23. Ridet JL, Malhotra SK, Privat A et al. (1997) Reactive astrocytes: cellular and molecular cues to biological function. Trends Neurosci 20: 570–7.

24. Sims TJ, Gilmore SA, Waxman SG (1991) Radial glia give rise to perinodal processes. Brain Res 549: 25–35.

25. Felts PA, Baker TA, Smith KJ (1997) Conduction in segmentally demyelinated mammalian central axons. J Neurosci 17: 7267–77.

26. Felts PA, Deecinek TJ, Ellisman MH et al. (1998) Sodium and potassium channel immunolocalisation in demyelinated and remyelinated central axons. Neuropathol Appl Neurobiol 24: 154–5.

27. Bostock H, Sears TA (1976) Continuous conduction in demyelinated mammalian nerve fibers. Nature 263: 786–7.

28. Craner MJ, Newcombe J, Black JA et al. (2004) Molecular changes in neurons in multiple sclerosis: altered axonal expression of Nav1.2 and Nav1.6 sodium channels and Na+/Ca2+ exchanger. Proc Natl Acad Sci USA 101: 8168–73.

29. Prineas JW, Connell F (1979) Remyelination in multiple sclerosis. Ann Neurol 5: 22–31.

30. Prineas JW, Barnard RO, Kwon EE et al. (1993) Multiple sclerosis: remyelination of nascent lesions. Ann Neurol 33: 137–51.

31. Smith KJ, Blakemore WF, McDonald WI (1981) The restoration of conduction by central remyelination. Brain 104: 383–404.

32. Felts PA, Smith KJ (1992) Conduction properties of central nerve fibers remyelinated by Schwann cells. Brain Res 574: 178–92.

33. Jeffery ND, Blakemore WF (1997) Locomotor deficits induced by experimental spinal cord demyelination are abolished by spontaneous remyelination. Brain 120: 27–37.

34. Jones SJ, Brusa A (2003) Neurophysiological evidence for long-term repair of MS lesions: implications for axon protection. J Neurol Sci 206: 193–8.

35. Frackowiak RS (1997) The cerebral basis of functional recovery. In: Frackowiak RS, Friston KJ, Frith CD et al., eds. Human Brain Function, 1st edn. Academic Press, San Diego: 275–99.

36. Grafman J, Litvan I (1999) Evidence for four forms of neuroplasticity. In: Grafman J, Christen Y, eds. Neuronal Plasticity: Building a bridge from the laboratory to the clinic (research and perspectives in neurosciences). Springer-Verlag, Berlin: 131–9.

37. Lotze M, Flor H, Grodd W et al. (2001) Phantom movements and pain. An fMRI study in upper limb amputees. Brain 124: 2268–77.

38. Wexler BE, Fulbright RK, Lacadie CM et al. (1997) An fMRI study of the human cortical motor system response to increasing functional demands. Magn Reson Imaging 15: 385–96.

39. Catalan MJ, Honda M, Weeks RA et al. (1998) The functional neuroanatomy of simple and complex sequential finger movements: a PET study. Brain 121: 253–64.

40. Ward NS, Frackowiak RS (2003) Age-related changes in the neural correlates of motor performance. Brain 126: 873–88.

41. Toosy A, Werring D, Bullmore E et al. (2002) Functional magnetic resonance imaging of the cortical response to photic stimulation in humans following optic neuritis recovery. Neurosci Lett 330: 255.

42. Russ MO, Cleff U, Lanfermann H et al. (2002) Functional magnetic resonance imaging in acute unilateral optic neuritis. J Neuroimaging 12: 339–50.

43. Werring DJ, Bullmore ET, Toosy AT et al. (2000) Recovery from optic neuritis is associated with a change in the distribution of cerebral response to visual stimulation: a functional magnetic resonance imaging study. J Neurol Neurosurg Psychiatry 68: 441–9.

44. Rombouts SA, Lazeron RH, Scheltens P et al. (1998) Visual activation patterns in patients with optic neuritis: an fMRI pilot study. Neurology 50: 1896–9.

45. Toosy AT, Hickman SJ, Plant GT et al. (2002) A longitudinal study of the cortical response to photic stimulation after acute optic neuritis using functional magnetic resonance imaging: a preliminary analysis. Ann Neurol 52[3S]: S41, abstract.

46. Toosy AT, Hickman SJ, Miszkiel KA et al. (2005) Adaptive cortical

plasticity in higher visual areas after acute optic neuritis. Ann Neurol 57: 622–33.

47. Rocca MA, Mezzapesa DM, Falini A et al. (2003) Evidence for axonal pathology and adaptive cortical reorganization in patients at presentation with clinically isolated syndromes suggestive of multiple sclerosis. Neuroimage 18: 847–55.

48. Pantano P, Iannetti GD, Caramia F et al. (2002) Cortical motor reorganization after a single clinical attack of multiple sclerosis. Brain 125: 1607–15.

49. Pantano P, Mainero C, Iannetti GD et al. (2002) Contribution of corticospinal tract damage to cortical motor reorganization after a single clinical attack of multiple sclerosis. Neuroimage 17: 1837–43.

50. Rocca MA, Mezzapesa DM, Ghezzi A et al. (2003) Cord damage elicits brain functional reorganization after a single episode of myelitis. Neurology 61: 1078–85.

51. Reddy H, Narayanan S, Matthews PM et al. (2000) Relating axonal injury to functional recovery in MS. Neurology 54: 236–9.

52. Lee MA, Blamire AM, Pendlebury S et al. (2000) Axonal injury or loss in the internal capsule and motor impairment in multiple sclerosis. Arch Neurol 57: 65–70.

53. Reddy H, Narayanan S, Arnoutelis R et al. (2000) Evidence for adaptive functional changes in the cerebral cortex with axonal injury from multiple sclerosis. Brain 123: 2314–20.

54. Reddy H, Narayanan S, Woolrich M et al. (2002) Functional brain reorganization for hand movement in patients with multiple sclerosis: defining distinct effects of injury and disability. Brain 125: 2646–57.

55. Mainero C, Caramia F, Pozzilli C et al. (2004) fMRI evidence of brain reorganization during attention and memory tasks in multiple sclerosis. Neuroimage 21: 858–67.

56. Staffen W, Mair A, Zauner H et al. (2002) Cognitive function and fMRI in patients with multiple sclerosis: evidence for compensatory cortical activation during an attention task. Brain 125: 1275–82.

57. Rocca MA, Gavazzi C, Mezzapesa DM et al. (2003) A functional magnetic resonance imaging study of patients with secondary progressive multiple sclerosis. Neuroimage 19: 1770–7.

58. Filippi M, Comi G (2002) Primary Progressive Multiple Sclerosis. Springer-Verlag, Milan.

59. Rocca MA, Matthews PM, Caputo D et al. (2002) Evidence of widespread movement-associated functional MRI changes in patients with PP MS. Neurology 58: 866–72.

60. Filippi M, Rocca MA, Falini A et al. (2002) Correlations between structural CNS damage and functional MRI changes in primary progressive MS. Neuroimage 15: 537–46.

61. Ciccarelli O, Toosy AT, Marsden JF et al. (2006) Functional response

to active and passive ankle movements with clinical correlations in patients with PP MS. J Neurol [Epub ahead of print].

62. Halliday AM, McDonald WI, Mushin J (1972) Delayed visual evoked response in optic neuritis. Lancet 1: 982–5.

63. Waxman SG (1981) Clinicopathological correlations in multiple sclerosis and related diseases. Adv Neurol 31: 169–82.

64. Perkin GD, Rose FC (1979) Optic Neuritis and its Differential Diagnosis. Oxford University Press, Oxford.

65. Hopper CL, Matthews CG, Cleeland CS (1972) Symptom instability and thermoregulation in multiple sclerosis. Neurology 22: 142–8.

66. Paintal AS (1966) The influence of diameter of medullated nerve fibres of cats on the rising and falling phases of the spike and its recovery. J Physiol 184: 791–811.

67. Davis FA, Schauf CL (1981) Approaches to the development of pharmacological interventions in multiple sclerosis. Adv Neurol 31: 505–10.

68. Smith KJ, McDonald WI (1980) Spontaneous and mechanically evoked activity due to central demyelinating lesion. Nature 286: 154–5.

69. Smith KJ, McDonald WI (1982) Spontaneous and evoked electrical discharges from a central demyelinating lesion. J Neurol Sci 55: 39–47.

70. Rizzo MA, Kocsis JD, Waxman SG (1996) Mechanisms of paresthesiae, dysesthesiae, and hyperesthesiae: role of Na+ channel heterogeneity. Eur Neurol 36: 3–12.

71. Kapoor R, Li YG, Smith KJ (1997) Slow sodium-dependent potential oscillations contribute to ectopic firing in mammalian demyelinated axons. Brain 120: 647–52.

72. Kapoor R, Smith KJ, Felts PA et al. (1993) Internodal potassium currents can generate ectopic impulses in mammalian myelinated axons. Brain Res 611: 165–9.

73. Davis FA, Bergen D, Schauf C et al. (1976) Movement phosphenes in optic neuritis: a new clinical sign. Neurology 26: 1100–4.

74. Ferguson B, Matyszak MK, Esiri MM et al. (1997) Axonal damage in acute multiple sclerosis lesions. Brain 120: 393–9.

75. Trapp BD, Peterson J, Ransohoff RM et al. (1998) Axonal transection in the lesions of multiple sclerosis. N Engl J Med 338: 278–85.

76. Perry VH, Anthony DC (1999) Axon damage and repair in multiple sclerosis. Philos Trans R Soc Lond B Biol Sci 354: 1641–7.

77. Trapp BD, Peterson J, Ransohoff RM et al. (1998) Axonal transection in the lesions of multiple sclerosis. N Engl J Med 338: 278–85.

78. Sadatipour BT, Greer JM, Pender MP (1998) Increased circulating antiganglioside antibodies in primary and secondary progressive multiple sclerosis. Ann Neurol 44: 980–3.

79. Smith KJ, Lassmann H (2002) The role of nitric oxide in multiple sclerosis. Lancet Neurol 1: 232–41.

80. Griffiths I, Klugmann M, Anderson T et al. (1998) Axonal swellings and degeneration in mice lacking the major proteolipid of myelin. Science 280: 1610–13.

81. Ganter P, Prince C, Esiri MM (1999) Spinal cord axonal loss in multiple sclerosis: a post-mortem study. Neuropathol Appl Neurobiol 25: 459–67.

82. Losseff NA, Webb SL, O'Riordan JI et al. (1996) Spinal cord atrophy and disability in multiple sclerosis. A new reproducible and sensitive MRI method with potential to monitor disease progression. Brain 119: 701–8.

83. Bermel RA, Bakshi R (2006) The measurement and clinical relevance of brain atrophy in multiple sclerosis. Lancet Neurol 5: 158–70.

84. Filippi M, Rocca MA, Comi G (2003) The use of quantitative magnetic-resonance-based techniques to monitor the evolution of multiple sclerosis. Lancet Neurol 2: 337–46.

85. Matthews PM, Pioro E, Narayanan S et al. (1996) Assessment of lesion pathology in multiple sclerosis using quantitative MRI morphometry and magnetic resonance spectroscopy. Brain 119: 715–22.

86. Fu L, Matthews PM, De Stefano N et al. (1998) Imaging axonal damage of normal-appearing white matter in multiple sclerosis. Brain 121: 103–13.

87. De Stefano N, Matthews PM, Fu L et al. (1998) Axonal damage correlates with disability in patients with relapsing–remitting multiple sclerosis. Results of a longitudinal magnetic resonance spectroscopy study. Brain 121: 1469–77.

88. Davie CA, Barker GJ, Webb S et al. (1995) Persistent functional deficit in multiple sclerosis and autosomal dominant cerebellar ataxia is associated with axon loss. Brain 118: 1583–92.

89. Dalton CM, Brex PA, Jenkins R et al. (2002) Progressive ventricular enlargement in patients with clinically isolated syndromes is associated with the early development of multiple sclerosis. J Neurol Neurosurg Psychiatry 73: 141–7.

90. Chard DT, Griffin CM, Parker GJ et al. (2002) Brain atrophy in clinically early relapsing–remitting multiple sclerosis. Brain 125: 327–37.

91. Hickman SJ, Brex PA, Brierley CM et al. (2001) Detection of optic nerve atrophy following a single episode of unilateral optic neuritis by MRI using a fat-saturated short-echo fast FLAIR sequence. Neuroradiology 43: 123–8.

92. Trip SA, Schlottmann PG, Jones SJ et al. (2005) Retinal nerve fiber layer axonal loss and visual dysfunction in optic neuritis. Ann Neurol 58: 383–91.

93. Smith KJ, Kapoor R, Hall SM et al. (2001) Electrically active axons degenerate when exposed to nitric oxide. Ann Neurol 49: 470–6.

94. Petzold A, Rejdak K, Plant GT (2004) Axonal degeneration and

inflammation in acute optic neuritis. J Neurol Neurosurg Psychiatry 75: 1178–80.

95. Lewis RA, Sumner AJ, Brown MJ et al. (1982) Multifocal demyelinating neuropathy with persistent conduction block. Neurology 32: 958–64.

96. Pluchino S, Quattrini A, Brambilla E et al. (2003) Injection of adult neurospheres induces recovery in a chronic model of multiple sclerosis. Nature 422: 688–94.

97. Pluchino S, Martino G (2005) The therapeutic use of stem cells for myelin repair in autoimmune demyelinating disorder. J Neurol Sci 233: 117–19.

2

The impact of living with multiple sclerosis: the need for a collaborative approach to care

Bernadette Porter, Ben Murphy and Charles Morland

Introduction

People with multiple sclerosis (MS) often come into contact with health and social care professionals when they are most vulnerable. Research shows that they would like to feel valued and cared for. In order to do this effectively health professionals need to examine their relationships with people with MS. In particular there is a need to ensure that the service offered is not one which does things to or for people but one which is collaborative, one which works with people to support their needs.

If health professionals are serious about delivering the best possible care then they must ensure that people with MS are treated with honesty, dignity and respect and talked to and listened to as an equal. This chapter aims to review some of the literature associated with the impact of living with MS but more importantly provides an insight into the reality of living with MS as shared by Ben and Charles.

To achieve collaboration we need to have a better understanding of how and when we can improve things. We need to actively listen to people who use our services and find out about their experience. We need to make sure that people have information to make choices, to feel confident and feel in control. We need to acknowledge each individual's expertise in managing their own life and recognize the small part that health professionals play. We need to see ourselves and services offered from a user's perspective as highlighted by Ben:

> It takes one sentence and probably 10 seconds to tell a person they have MS... and a lifetime to deal with it.

> You can measure the health professional's input in hours, my life is in years.

It is truly important that we explore beyond our professional silos and challenge our approach to care delivery. When we are in contact with a person with MS we need to ask whether the person with MS is getting the best care, in the right place from the right person or team. If the answer is no then we must endeavor to correct things. In addition to challenging how we work we need to recognize the wealth of knowledge people with MS accumulate whilst living with the disease. We need to create opportunities for shared learning within expert patient and health professional arenas. As a person living with a long disability Charles remarked:

> Long-term disability of people who are neither dying nor getting better is boring. The only people passionately interested are the long term disabled themselves; make use of them.

It is hoped that this chapter enlightens you on the impact of MS and inspires health and social care professionals to invite people with MS to share their knowledge within educational, discussion, service planning and developmental arenas.

Introduction to Ben and Charles

Ben

I am 34 years old, a chartered accountant, live in London, and have Relapsing Remitting Multiple Sclerosis.

In February of 2002 I began to experience double vision, my right eye being unable to move beyond the center of my line of vision. After several visits to an ophthalmologist following referral by my GP, and sporting an elegant pair of pink prism spectacles, I became aware that I couldn't walk properly, and kept on losing my balance with my legs becoming weak and unresponsive.

I was lucky enough to have private medical insurance with my employer, and I made an appointment with who I thought was the consultant neurologist for Maundy Thursday 2002. I was assured by the consultant urologist that it wasn't the first time confusion had arisen and it wouldn't be the last.

I spent the Easter weekend with my family and friends in Liverpool not knowing what was happening to me, and in a worrying state of limbo, as my symptoms were still quite extreme, especially given that I had had no previous indications of a problem until this time. From being a physically active, sporty young man to this state was incomprehensible. I am fortunate to have a strong family network, and at this worrying time I found their support invaluable.

The following week I saw the consultant neurologist who arranged an MRI scan of my brain, and within a week I had a firm diagnosis of MS. At that instant I was relieved, a weight lifted from my mind. My worst fears were not realized, as I had thought of several worse eventualities, such as an aneurism or even a brain tumor. I had a fair idea that MS wasn't a fatal condition, and could even be managed. In fact I felt mildly elated that with this diagnosis I could move forward after 2 months of uncertainty and panic.

My eyesight had cleared up by this point, but I couldn't walk without the support of an umbrella. I was given 3 days intra-venous methyl-prednisolone (IVMP), a potent corticosteroid. The results were spectacular, and it was as if nothing had happened, my walking and balance restored to their 'pre-attack' state.

Charles

I was diagnosed with MS aged 43 in 1983. The first symptom was a numbness in a finger. My GP referred me to a specialist in Harley Street and after various tests culminating in a lumbar puncture the diagnosis was confirmed within six months.

At an early stage, I experienced a numbness of one side of my face, but that recovered within weeks and since then the disability is concentrated in my legs combined with insensitivity and clumsiness in my hand and fingers. Deterioration has been gradual without sudden relapses or remissions. I began using a wheel-chair in 1994 and now use it constantly, although I can still stand to shave and dress. I live without any 'care' support and lived on my own for seven years.

When I was diagnosed in 1983 neither I nor my family (a wife and two teenage sons) knew anything of, nor anyone with, MS. The neurologist made his diagnosis efficiently. He provided little information about the likely progression of the disease and no advice about available support when I took my wife with me to the final meeting.

In these circumstances my wife and I decided that we would tell no one about my condition except our sons aged 14 and 16. In retrospect this was the wrong decision. It put unnecessary pressure on all of us while what we needed was the support of our wider family and friends. This we received unstintingly as soon as the situation became public.

Background

The mean age of multiple sclerosis onset is 20–40 years. The diagnosis and symptoms frequently coincide with important milestones and transition stages in the person's family life.[1] The psychosocial impact of MS can be vast, effecting patients and their families in a myriad of ways including loss of income, employment issues, impact on relationships, impact on parental roles, emotional burden and adjustment difficulties.[2]

Although MS can have devastating effects on an individual's level of function it has relatively little effect on life expectancy and may have to be managed for many decades. The diagnosis impacts on all aspects of life and people with MS may need to make extensive use of health and social services. People with MS must be supported to become experts to influence and self-manage key aspects of their care pathway. An important tool to optimize self-management is the empowerment of patients through expert patient programs.[3] There is a growing body of evidence that approaches to management of chronic illness which incorporate the patient as a co-partner in care, demonstrates improved outcomes.[4] Areas of improvements have included reduced severity of symptoms, significant decrease in pain, improved life control and activity, and improved resourcefulness and life satisfaction.[5]

As people with MS will often have several problems that need resolution by input from a number of professionals, effective teamwork, communication and co-ordination is essential to optimize goal orientated management plans. In addition to assessment of physical aspects of the disease, the assessment of psychosocial issues is an integral component in the comprehensive care and management of patients with MS.[6] The health professional's approach to delivery of service is another essential component in support of self-management strategies. As MS is unpredictable, services need to be designed so that they are flexible, timely and responsive, encouraging self-referral and appropriate assessment by team members.[7] Essential components of good long-term disease management are summarized in Box 2.1.[8]

Impact of diagnosis

The diagnostic phase has been highlighted as a crucial time for people with MS and has been described as a period of anxious

---

Box 2.1. Essential components of good team approach to long-term disease management.

- Involving people in their own care
- Coordinating care
- Multidisciplinary teamwork
- Integration of specialist and generalist expertise including cross-boundary working
- Minimizing unnecessary visits and admissions
- Providing care in the least intensive setting

Box 2.2. Key issues for people at time of diagnosis[13]

- Certain, clear diagnosis
- Appropriate support at diagnosis
- Access to information
- Continuing education

waiting. The delay between presentation of symptoms, diagnostic tests and receipt of results is a recurring area of complaint.[9–11] The care received at the time of diagnosis is central to the adaptation processes as information given and received may impact on the person with MS for the rest of their life.[12] Appropriate support, information, education and guidance can help people adapt to the impact of the diagnosis. People with MS want a clear, accurate diagnosis, access to appropriate support, information and continuing education at and around the time of diagnosis[13] (Box 2.2)

Research has shown that the newly diagnosed person may have a multitude of needs, including living with an uncertain future, experiencing wide symptomatic variability and needing emotional, spiritual and psychosocial support. Specialist MS nurses and allied health professionals are well placed to provide support at this crucial time. A model of care that summarizes

Box 2.3. Support at time of diagnosis[14]

E = Education
     (about the disease, its course, symptomatic management and
     psychosocial implications)
A = Adaptation
     (adjustment, modifying lifestyle, setting priorities, promoting
     self-care)
S = Support
     (counseling, providing information on support groups, help in
     obtaining entitlements)
E = Enhancement
     (self-care, improvement of coping skills, facilitation of
     communication about needs and concerns

what a patient and their family need during this difficult time is given in Box 2.3.[14]

By provision of clear, accurate evidence-based information the patient and their families can feel informed and supported. This approach can be initiated at the time of diagnosis through information sessions. The health professional can listen to fears and worries, assess the patient's perception of the disease, correct misconceptions, explain the pathology of existing symptoms and make appropriate referrals to meet individual needs. It is important to recognize that physical function, social interaction and emotional wellbeing can affect how the person with MS and their family cope and adapt to the diagnosis. By understanding the impact of the diagnosis the health professional can introduce the concept of self-management to the person with MS.

Charles' thoughts on management of the diagnostic phase

The major minus of coping on our own was the lack of practical information about MS and the absence of any knowledgeable moral support. Every neurologist who regularly delivers the bleak diagnosis of an incurable and unpredictable disease should, in my view, as a matter of course find the time to discuss the implications with the patient and take the initiative in including family members in the discussion as a matter of routine. Even more important for me and my family would have been the opportunity to meet others with a similar diagnosis and see how they lived and survived. Here again the neurologist should take the initiative with his new patient and identify suitable volunteers from his other patients who could be telephoned or visited. This would not be difficult.

Ben's tips to newly diagnosed

If I was to summarize a plan of attack for the newly-diagnosed, I would find it difficult not to paraphrase clichés, but there is considerable hope and potential around.

- It is important to listen to your body and become expert in how you feel

- Keep talking to MS professionals, as they have seen thousands of people at various stages of the disease, and the sufferer can only draw from one life
- Look for a simple life, as far as is possible
- Respect the disease, and give it enough time in the day
- Plan your day and indeed your life, allowing you to identify problems and issues which need to be dealt with
- Remember everybody is only too willing to help
- Steer clear of the internet; use only information sites recommended by MS professionals; a Google search for 'MS' brings up some worrying scenarios, which may not happen to you

Encouraging self-management

The majority of people with MS want to be involved in their overall management plan; however, they must be supported to do so. There is evidence that the quality of communication at the time of diagnosing a chronic disease influences patient health outcomes.[15] Good history taking and discussion of management plans have been found to have positive effects on emotional health, symptom resolution, general functioning, physiological measures and pain control.[15] In addition to good communication, people with MS require timely, accurate information and support. Education and support are an ongoing part of management from diagnosis to enable individuals to actively participate in their own care.

Ben's quest to actively manage the disease

As 2002 progressed and moved into early summer, I enjoyed what I look upon now as almost a honeymoon period. I was armed with a diagnosis of MS, and was literally walking tall with the knowledge that if I was to suffer another attack, steroids would put me back on my feet.

A relapse in June, followed by one in August, both treated with steroids, let me know that I was in for the long haul and my happy state of mind that all could be solved with steroids necessarily changed. It became evident that I would have to address some fundamental issues which up to then I had been oblivious of/ignored.

Another relapse at the end of September could not be resolved with steroids as it would have been too soon following the previous doses. A new approach had to be taken to my condition and in November 2002 my GP referred me to a specialist center.

The holistic approach of the MS specialist center was nothing short of inspirational and was a revelation to me, as the private neurologist I had been seeing up to that point had said that there was not much else he could do for me.

People with MS are often expert in detecting and anticipating changes in their health and wellbeing. Health and social care professionals should support people with MS to become expert

Box 2.4. Requirements to self-manage a chronic disease[16]

- Knowing how to recognize and act upon symptoms
- Dealing with acute attacks of the disease
- Making effective use of treatments/medicines
- Comprehending the implications of professional advice
- Establishing a sleep pattern and dealing with fatigue
- Assessing social and other services
- Managing work
- Accessing leisure activities
- Developing strategies to deal with the psychological impact of the illness
- Learning to cope with other people's response to their illness

Box 2.5. Five core self-management skills in managing a chronic illness[16]

Self management skills
- Problem solving
- Decision making
- Resource utilization
- Formation of patient/health professional partnership
- Action taking

patients by aiming to give the person the knowledge, skills and confidence to participate actively in all aspects of their own care.[4] The key requirements to self-management of a chronic condition are summarized in Box 2.4, whilst the core skills necessary are summarized in Box 2.5.[16]

Charles' views on expertise

The experts living with MS are those who have it and have had it for many years. The health professionals should ensure that they are involved in every aspect of diagnosis and subsequent support as well as in the training of the professionals themselves and the selection and installation of equipment for the disabled.

Making use of this largely wasted pool of experience and expertise would also give great satisfaction to those with MS and also go some way towards combating another major obstacle. My experience is that, because I am in a wheelchair, people presume, at least initially, that I am mentally disabled as well. Questions are addressed to the upright companion and conversation take place literally over my head. This happens as often in doctors' surgeries and hospitals as it does in shops and airports.

Key areas of concern to people living with MS

Assessment of new or increased symptoms

In terms of relapses, people should be given information regarding general health factors, such as infection, that may influence the risk of relapse, and be advised how to detect relapses and what to do if new symptoms occur, including how to self-refer into primary or secondary care clinics.

In the event of new or increased symptoms, people with MS should be able to identify and contact a professional from their healthcare team who can advise them or direct them to the most appropriate local service. If a person with MS develops new or increased neurological symptoms a formal assessment should be made to determine the diagnosis. At the assessment the possibility of any other medical cause for an increase in neurological symptoms must be considered. In particular it is important to exclude an infective cause such as a urinary tract infection, which may be otherwise clinically silent. The possibility of dual neurological pathology – for example, a cord compression mimicking a spinal cord relapse – should also be borne in mind.[17] If the new symptoms are assessed to be unrelated to MS it must still be ensured that the person with MS has access to the appropriate service and treatment.

Ben's relapses

I have had seven disabling relapses. There appears to be no rhyme or reason to their onset.

A relapse for me begins with an uncomfortable, uneasy feeling all over my body. This does not necessarily mean that a relapse is inevitable as it can dissipate during the course of a day, but it is an indication of what may come.

If, then, my legs become stiff, and do not do what I ask of them, and I find myself concentrating harder than usual on walking and balancing, and I become very reliant on my walking stick, and if this is maintained over the course of three to four days, then I can be pretty sure that I am embarking on a prolonged exacerbation of my MS symptoms, AKA a relapse.

To a certain extent, I diagnose my own relapses, as it is only me who knows how I feel and understands my relative disability. A relapse to me means several things, which can be divided into physical and mental aspects.

Physical impact of Ben's relapse

My legs become unresponsive, and my feet catch on the smallest of obstructions, and I cannot walk without extreme effort, concentration and difficulty.

At my worst I feel as if I am walking through ever thickening syrup, and I can't walk 50 yards even with a walking stick.

I need to concentrate very hard on apparently simple tasks such as making a cup of tea. The concentration needed can be very draining, and leads to exhaustion.

Getting to work is practically difficult if not impossible, public transport becoming daunting and forbidding, especially rush hour tube journeys. A flight of stairs without a banister is like a brick wall to me. Even with a banister stairs are a considerable hurdle.

My sense of balance comes from my vision, more so during a period of relapse and if there is too much going on around me it can lead to a stumble or even a fall, viz busy London railway stations.

My day-to-day routine has to change, and I need to become exceptionally organized and regimented. A relapse can also bin any short term plans I may have had, as an inability to walk overshadows pretty much everything else in my life. This can and has been upsetting and disappointing.

Mental impact of Ben's relapse

I don't find that the physical aspects of a relapse upset me, but what does is the thought process which my brain takes me through. 'Was there anything I did wrong?' 'Should I have done things differently?' 'Was it something I ate or drank?', 'did I overdo it?', and a great deal of soul-searching must happen, which is only human nature.

The psychological aspects have for me been more diffi-cult to deal with. My overbearing feeling when a relapse comes on is not misery or depression, but the worry that this could be the relapse which leaves permanent damage and disability, or puts me in a wheelchair.

These thoughts can be fatalistic, and are of course unrealistic, but they are always at the back of my mind and it can be tough to stay focused and to lift one's head from the fog and confusion of the short-term situation.

Early relapses induced a 'why me?' feeling, which I think is only natural when you cannot understand what is happen-ing to your body; it is also quite tough to comprehend the relative disability compared to even the previous day or week, when I had been metaphorically running and jumping around.

The unpredictability of the onset and duration of relapses can be frustrating. I missed a wedding of a good friend in

July 2004 due to a particularly ferocious relapse. I'd been looking forward to meeting old friends from school, who probably wouldn't get together again in one group.

With RRMS, you learn to live with such irritations, for that is all they are. Initially it felt to me as if I couldn't plan for anything, but to quote the school teacher from South Park, 'Life ain't fair, kiddo, get used to it.' That said, my overall outlook doesn't change, but any short term plans I may have had are put on hold for a while.

Comprehensive multidisciplinary management of relapse

An acute relapse is an episode of neurological disturbance, of the kind seen in MS, that lasts for at least 24 hours, and for which there is no other cause such as fever.[18] Typically a relapse evolves over a few days, reaches a plateau, and then remits to a variable degree over a few weeks or months. The patient experiencing a relapse has to cope with a comparatively sudden onset of neurological symptoms that may be physically and psychologically distressing and functionally and socially incapacitating. In the longer term, incomplete remission from a relapse may result in residual neurological deficit. Management of an acute relapse requires a comprehensive approach addressing its medical, functional and psychosocial effects. Management incorporates education regarding relapses, support in the event of a relapse, treatment to accelerate or improve the recovery from a relapse, and symptomatic treatment and rehabilitation.

Ben's experience of dealing with a relapse

I have two options at the outset of a relapse. I can telephone the center, and attend the relapse clinic, where a neurologist assesses whether intravenous methylprednisolone (IVMP) would be appropriate. If I am offered steroids, and I have decided that this is the best plan of attack, a 3-day course of IVMP follows, which involves attending hospital. There is a move afoot for home visits, which in my opinion is ideal as when I am at my least able, I need to tackle public transport etc. to get to hospital.

Whilst being aware that I am lucky in having the intravenous steroid option, I don't always take that route. I sometimes prefer to sit the relapse out. This requires not a small amount of resolve and mental strength but has in the past meant absence from work for four weeks, which is not ideal.

Whether I choose the steroid option depends on what else is happening in my life, what my work situation is and what I need to be able to do. My coping mechanism has become fine tuned over the past 4 years, and an overriding frame of mind when in the midst of a relapse is to remember that it is more likely that it isn't a permanent state of affairs.

At the back of my mind I know that steroids are not a long term solution, but a temporary fix to hopefully a temporary problem. Another aspect I think about when considering relapse management is if I decide to take the steroid option I will be in close contact with the specialist team. It is comforting to be in an arena where everybody understands my situation and where advice, treatment and support is available. Knowing that this service is available to me is empowering and humbling.

Management of acute relapses should not just be limited to corticosteroid therapy but should be comprehensive, tackling all aspects of the relapse. Practical supportive measures, such as the provision of care or equipment, may be essential and should not be forgotten. Symptomatic treatment for new symptoms from a relapse may sometimes be required. If a relapse is improving spontaneously or with corticosteroids the duration of symptoms may be too short to warrant symptomatic treatment. However, if symptoms are distressing or not resolving then treatment may be required. Symptomatic treatments are not discussed further here but are covered in Chapter 4.

Functional recovery from a relapse may be facilitated by multidisciplinary input from neurological rehabilitation services. This input should run in parallel with any medical treatment and depending on need may be on an outpatient or inpatient basis. A recent randomized controlled trial found a multidisciplinary rehabilitation approach to be superior to a standard ward routine in people with MS receiving intravenous corticosteroid therapy.[19] Inpatient rehabilitation has also been shown to be useful in relapsing–remitting MS particularly in people with incomplete recovery from relapses with moderate to severe disability.[20]

Diet

Many people with MS are concerned about the impact of MS on lifestyle and are interested in finding out about the role of diet in maintenance of health. There is no substantial evidence to support special diets such as gluten-free; however, many people incorporate such diets into their self-management plans. People often ask whether alcohol is contraindicated. There is no evidence that moderate intake of alcohol affects MS disease activity, although it may impact on urinary symptoms (it is a bladder irritant) or exacerbate balance, mobility or speech problems. It is advisable to check if alcohol is contraindicated with some prescribed medications. A daily intake of 1.5 liters of water is advised for maintenance of health.

The role of essential fatty acids in MS has been researched with some evidence suggesting that omega-6 linolic acid may benefit people with MS. Although there is still some debate about the exact role of essential fatty acids in MS there is agreement that linoleic acid is an important element of a healthy diet. In the UK, NICE guidelines advise that an intake of 17–23 g per day of linoleic acid may slow down the disabling effects of MS.[21]

Overall, in the absence of allergy and intolerance, people with MS should be advised that a diet balanced with low saturated fats, carbohydrates and 'five a day' fruit or vegetables is recommended. People should be made aware that the occasional treat that is high in saturated fat, sugar or salt will not cause harm and that a well-balanced diet should cover all nutritional requirements, without need for nutritional supplements.[22]

People with MS who are over- or underweight or have symptoms that interfere with eating or swallowing should be referred to appropriate team members, including dietitians, speech and language therapists, nurses and occupational therapists, for advice and support to optimize dietary and fluid intake.

Ben's thoughts on diet

In the summer of 2004 I thought I had found the answer to life, after I had my blood tested for food intolerances. I genuinely felt that after discovering I had a horrific intolerance to cow's milk and egg white I had solved all my problems.

It was as if a dense fog had lifted and I could see an aspect of MS which I could control. Every Saturday and Sunday morning I'd been having bacon and eggs for my breakfast and my walking was shocking. I stopped eating eggs and taking milk in my tea and the effect was immediate. I began to keep a detailed diet diary, with a view to highlighting any other intolerances I may have.

This didn't of course change the fact that I had MS, but was one of two things (along with exercise) which had a real and tangible effect on my life.

Fatigue

Fatigue can be one of the most common, disabling and frustrating symptoms experienced by a person with MS. People with MS ranked fatigue as one of the MS-related symptoms that most impaired their quality of life.[23] The presence of fatigue may vary widely between people with MS and within a person from time to time. Fatigue is associated with disability and depression and it can be difficult to distinguish the impact of fatigue from other symptoms. It is important that healthcare professionals recognize fatigue when it is present, assessing whether it is a significant problem in a person's life. Mood, disturbed sleep and current medications should be assessed to analyze whether they are primary or symptomatic in nature. Referral to specialist occupational therapists for advice and training on how to manage fatigue including advice on aerobic exercise and energy conservation techniques should be offered, whilst some individuals report benefit from drugs such as amantadine.

Exercise

People with MS are often afraid to participate in exercise programs as they are afraid that they may exacerbate the disease or cause problems. This may be related to past experience of symptoms such as tingling or Uthoff's phenomenon. Healthcare professionals should take time to explain the mechanisms associated with short circuiting of signals and temporary symptoms associated with raised temperature in order to allay concerns.

People with MS should be made aware that there is now clear evidence that they benefit from exercise programs and that people with MS respond to exercise the same way as those without MS: they become more fit.[24] Studies have shown that those who engage in aerobic exercise improve aerobic fitness, those engaged in resistive training improve strength and those who engage in respiratory exercises improve respiratory fitness levels.[25–27] None of the studies indicated a correlation between exercise and manifestation of relapse or disease activity. Whist there are a number of unanswered questions regarding exercise dosages and regimes for people with more advanced disease, health professionals should arrange assessments with specialist physiotherapists and encourage exercise as part of wellbeing and self-management programs.

Ben's thoughts on exercise

In 2003 I began to use a rowing machine 3 or 4 times per week. At the time I had no other feasible way of exercising, and after a couple of months I found I could row strenuously for 20 minutes at a time.

Swimming has now replaced the rowing, as I recently moved next door to a leisure center, and I swim 3 or 4 times per week for 45 minutes at a time. The feeling of well-being after exercise is wonderful, and it somehow clears my head in order that I can concentrate on important matters and not worry about the minutiae of life.

Vocational activities

People with MS are often well-educated and skilled workers with extensive employment histories, who constitute a valuable labor resource for the societies in which they live.[28]

Charles

At the time of diagnosis, I was a director of a big investment bank in the City and four years later I moved on to become

Chief Executive of a medium sized US owned investment bank. It was known when I was hired that I had MS.

After three years the demands of the job, which involved UK and US working hours and frequent trans-Atlantic travel, combined with some deterioration in my physical mobility, compelled me to retire as CEO. I continued in banking at a rather slower pace and became Chairman of a small new bank which was subsequently taken over.

At this time I became involved with Leonard Cheshire, a major charity working with disabled people, and following the death of my wife from cancer, became Chairman in 2000. My role, though non-executive, took up to two to three days a week overseeing Leonard Cheshire activities in the UK, where there are 150 centres working with 25,000 disabled people and employing 8000 staff; in addition, I travelled extensively, visiting operations in 30 of the 60 countries where we were represented. I retired after five years as Chairman in 2005.

At diagnosis most people with MS are in full-time education or employment; however, many leave work. A recent audit report from a large UK neurology center demonstrated that most people with MS are in employment at diagnosis, but that employment loss starts shortly after diagnosis with 80% of people with MS unemployed within 10 years of diagnosis.[29] The reasons for unemployment have not been clearly delineated and may be related to the disease itself, or to the working environment and demands of the job.[30,31]

The need to integrate health and employment teams to improve vocational rehabilitation is now well recognized. In the UK key documents highlight that people with long-term neurological conditions are to have access to appropriate vocational assessment, rehabilitation and ongoing support to enable them to find, regain or remain in work and access other occupational and educational opportunities.[32] Rehabilitation teams should offer services that provide mechanisms for people with MS to make adjustments in their careers and to continue working as long as they wish to. As an interdisciplinary exercise, vocational rehabilitation should blend the expertise of health professionals in psychology, counseling, social work, technology, human resources and law. Early intervention is key to supporting and training people to enable them to obtain, maintain and advance in jobs that are compatible with their interests, abilities and experience.

> ## Ben
>
> My line manager at work has been very supportive, and agreed to my request for a flexible working pattern. To avoid the crowds I get to work for 7.30 am, and this generally allows me to leave at 4–4.30, again avoiding the melee of London public transport at 'rush hour'.

MS is covered by the Disability Discrimination Act (DDA) from the point of diagnosis in many countries. In the UK the DDA prohibits unlawful discrimination in all aspects of employment – in recruitment, selection, training promotion, redundancy and dismissal, and places a duty on employers to make reasonable adjustments to the workplace or working arrangements (Box 2.6).[33] In the UK an Access to Work Scheme is available through disability employment advisors at Job Centre Plus offices who can offer advice about adjustments, grants and physical adaptations.

Pregnancy

The effect of pregnancy on disease activity is an important concern among young women.

> **Box 2.6.** Reasonable adjustments to facilitate employment[33]
>
> - Allocating some of your work to someone else
> - Transferring you to another post or another place of work
> - Making adjustments to the buildings where you work
> - Being flexible about your hours – allowing you to have different core working hours and to be away from the office for assessment, treatment or rehabilitation
> - Providing training
> - Providing modified equipment
> - Making instructions and manuals more accessible
> - Providing a reader or interpreter

A prospective study of pregnancy in MS confirmed that relapse rate declines during pregnancy, especially in the third trimester, increases during the first 3 months postpartum, and then returns to the pre-pregnancy rate.[34] In the same study epidural analgesia and breast feeding did not increase the risk of relapse. There is therefore no medical contraindication to pregnancy in MS. Women should be encouraged to seek medical advice before conception in order to review any medications and make changes as necessary. None of the disease-modifying drugs are considered safe during pregnancy and should be stopped, ideally in advance of conception. Disease-modifying drugs may be restarted following delivery if the mother does not plan to breast feed, otherwise treatment can be resumed once breast feeding is stopped. There are no contraindications to using analgesia, including transcutaneous nerve stimulation or epidural pain relief, during child birth.[35]

Sexual function

Like many symptoms, sexual dysfunction may or may not occur in MS, is impossible to predict and may occur for varying periods of time. When sexual dysfunction does occur it is mainly associated with impaired sexual physiology. In addition, impairments such as spasms may make sexual activity difficult, which may make it problematic for the person to establish or maintain partnership relations. Sexual dysfunction may be manifested as erectile and/or ejaculatory dysfunction in males, and loss of libido, loss of vaginal tone, painful heightened vaginal sensation and loss of ability to orgasm in females.

Health professionals should appreciate the private and intimate nature of discussing sexual function. People with MS should be asked sensitively about or given the opportunity to remark upon any difficulties that they may be having in establishing and/or maintaining wanted sexual and personal relationships and should be offered information about locally available counseling and supportive services. It is deemed good practice to offer every person or couple with persisting sexual dysfunction an opportunity to see a specialist with particular interest in sexual problems associated with neurological disease. Drug treatment may prove effective for males; however, there is no effective drug treatment for females with sexual dysfunction. Information leaflets with advice on body mapping, lubricants and the use of sexual aids[36] should be made available.

Family issues

MS has been described as 'the uninvited guest' in family life.[37] As MS is unpredictable, individuals with MS and their family members face challenges in planning and anticipating daily activities. Creativity and flexibility is often required to distribute the resources of time, energy and emotions appropriately among all family members.

Charles' thoughts on relationships

Because my disability has grown gradually, I have, until last year, had no reason to contact care professionals and it has been up to me and my family to devise ways of coping with my deteriorating physical capabilities. This has both advantages and disadvantages.

On the plus side it has retained my independence and control of how I live and what I do. An essential to achieving this was the refusal of my wife and sons to treat me as an invalid. They did not bring me my slippers or pat my head, although they were always there when it was really needed.

Another thing I was slow to grasp was that people, be they friends or strangers, not only are prepared to help but get positive pleasure and satisfaction from helping someone who needs it. The key is to ask while making it quite clear what help is required. I have also learned to accept when help is offered even when not really needed. Asking requires a certain amount of courage as well as swallowing one's pride.

The person with MS and their family may experience feelings of loss and grief with every new symptom and change in functional ability. MS can impact on a family's rhythm of carrying out daily routines and disruption in communication. People with MS may have difficulty describing unseen silent symptoms whilst family members may become overprotective resulting in unexpressed feelings.

Ben's thoughts on relationships

As I go through life, I have found that most people are nice. Sometimes I feel I'm asking for someone to do something which for me would be virtually impossible or hazardous, for example changing a ceiling light bulb, but I find that they are only too pleased to help. I have no concept that it is easy for them.

Of my family and friends, not one individual has changed in their approach or behavior towards me. They have all been a source of strength and comfort, and by the same token a levelling and normalizing influence when I occasionally become introvert and begin to feel sorry for myself.

It is acknowledged that parents frequently try to protect their children by not telling them anything, especially if there are few physical symptoms evident, believing that their own worries and anxieties do not show.[38] There is now evidence that a parent's level of 'invisible' symptoms of mood and anxiety impact negatively on children of people with MS.[39] Lack of open discussion can cause uncertainty and fear and may also discourage children from asking questions and talking about matters important to them. By contrast, open communication encourages honesty and a shared approach to facing the challenges as a family, which can help the child to cope. Teenagers of people with MS are at risk of taking on too much care and practical responsibilities. Health professionals should be aware of this, encouraging use of resources to support and minimize burden. The delivery of educational program models such as 'MS in the family workshops' can help facilitate discussion and open channels of communication, providing a safe environment for children of people with MS to share their concerns and learn from each other.[40]

Carers are people who help with the physical, emotional and daily needs of people who cannot manage all these activities on their own. Carers can be paid professionals but many carers are family members who provide emotional support, help with daily tasks, chores and intimate help. Many family members adjust very well to the caring role; however, there is evidence that caring can have a detrimental impact on a carer's psychological wellbeing. A detrimental impact on the psychological wellbeing status of partners and caregivers has been demonstrated in a number of studies.[41-43] One of the biggest conflicts that carers

Box 2.7. Assessment of family issues (adapted from reference 50)

- Assess family support system
- Assess family understanding and knowledge of MS
- Assess family coping behaviors and problem-solving techniques
- Assess impact of MS on parental role
- Assess impact of caring role on children
- Assess family activities and financial resources
- Assess impact and perceived impact of MS on family roles
- Assess family interactions and communication including expression of emotions
- Assess need to refer to appropriate support resources

face is the need to work in order to meet essential family needs, resulting in frustration, exhaustion and burnout. Studies have also shown that caregivers experience low levels of perceived social support[44,45] and have a low uptake of formal community support services.[46–49]

Healthcare teams should be aware of the impact of MS on family dynamics and should not overlook these issues when making assessments. It is important that health professionals employ sensitive, skilful assessment techniques of key areas (Box 2.7), ensuring appropriate referral to available resources.

Mood and emotional issues

Living with MS poses a number of challenges that can affect the way a person feels about themselves. It is not uncommon for people with MS to experience uncertainty, anxiety, poor self image, and feelings of grief and stress.[50] Living with MS presents a

Box 2.8. Challenges of daily life with MS (adapted from reference 51)

- Living with uncertainty
- Being informed – in charge
- Making personal decisions
- Balancing hope and realistic expectations
- Dealing with stress

number of challenges on a daily basis, as summarized in Box 2.8.[51] Health professionals can help support people with MS by providing support and education within an empowerment model, so that the person gains a sense of control and is able to participate actively in healthcare decisions and self-management strategies.

Ben: making personal decisions

I find I am keenly on the lookout for opportunities to make life simpler, and I do not let the condition interfere with my life, whilst paying it the attention it sometimes draws.

In late 2004, I became aware of a development in a part of London I'd previously lived in and enjoyed. I put a deposit down, and moved in in August 2005. A leisure center with a 25 meter swimming pool was also being built in the development, and this added up to a superb opportunity not to be missed.

I left a 2 bedroom house for a 1 bed flat, but the flat is low maintenance, I need only to walk 50 yards to get to the pool. I need not be a slave to the train timetable, and this has given my life more independence and flexibility.

Mood swings may include emotional lability, and uncontrollable laughter or crying may occur. Depression and anxiety (see Chapter 4) respond well to appropriate treatment; however, they are often not assessed. Reported rates of depression range from 10% to 57%[52] whilst rates of anxiety have been reported at 25%. These psychological manifestations may arise specific to neurological lesions or may be secondary to disability, altered life circumstances, pain or loss of employment. Health and social care providers have a particular opportunity to decrease depression-related morbidity and mortality. However, unfortunately they too often fail to identify, diagnose and treat mood disorders appropriately.[53–55] Given that suicide is more common among patients with MS than in both the general population[56] and patients with other neurological conditions, prompt diagnosis and successful treatment are particularly critical.[57,58]

The presence of depression and anxiety impacts on all aspects of life including family relationships.[59,60] A recent study that measured the impact of chronic parental illness on adolescent and adult children demonstrated levels of depression three times higher within children of people with MS than that seen in the normal population. Children of people with MS report lower scores in all dimensions of quality of life (QoL) when compared to children of parents with Parkinson's disease. Highly significant correlations were observed between the people with MS in QoL and mental wellbeing and the QoL of the child, a finding not seen in children of parents with Parkinson's disease. Results suggest that the impact on the child of parental Parkinson's disease is closely linked to the parent's ability to perform activities of daily living, whereas the impact of parental MS is significantly linked to the parent's emotional wellbeing.[39] MS also has a detrimental impact on the psychological wellbeing status of partners and caregivers as demonstrated in a number of studies.[61,62]

Disability and disease progression

People with MS who develop disability and disease progression face a number of challenges. Issues present at the time of minimal impairment such as role as parent, employment options and symptom management may become even more complex and challenging.

Disease progression is usually associated with loss of abilities, activities and life roles which activates grief and need for adaptation. People may need support to identify new goals and make different plans. The need for support and counseling at this period is as important as counseling at time of diagnosis and should not be ignored. People may be called upon to make important life decisions at a time when they may feel least equipped to do so.[63] Healthcare professionals should help people plan for problems or limitations so that important decisions can be made with deliberation rather than being forced upon at time of crisis.[63]

Management of these areas requires an integrated multidisciplinary approach that aims to reduce limitation in activities and restriction in participations, and improve QoL.[63]

Charles' thoughts on adaptation

The presumption of mental incapacity underlies a great deal of recent health and safety legislation. If a disabled person is of sound mind, then his freedom of action and of risk taking should be no more constrained than any other sane human being. Recent legislation appears to be driven more by the need to protect institutions and their staff from criticism and litigation and ignores the great damage to freedom of choice and independence of the disabled. Health professionals should use the maximum of common sense in their interpretation.

The key issues for people with moderate disability have been identified, as summarized in Box 2.9, whilst key issues for people with severe disability are summarized in Box 2.10.

Box 2.9. Key themes for people in moderate disability phase.[63] Recommendations on rehabilitation services for persons with multiple sclerosis in Europe

---

1. Responsiveness to needs related to significant changes in ability and accrued impairment
2. Access to and choice of different professional services
3. Access to multidisciplinary expertise in symptom and disability management and treatment
4. Communication and co-ordination between service providers and care agencies
5. Empowerment of persons with MS and their carers to enable them to take a partnership role in disease management and treatment

---

Mobility aids

People with MS who experience mobility loss should be offered expert advice on assistive technology devices. Wheeled mobility devices such as wheelchairs or scooters can offer a great deal of freedom and independence; however, proper selection is more complex than choosing from a catalog or specialist shop.[64] All health professionals of the MS team have a responsibility to understand the basics of device selection so that they can provide appropriate guidance and information. Assessment by specialist seating and mobility experts offers the best possible outcome.

> **Box 2.10.** Key themes for people in severe disability phase.[63]
> Recommendations on rehabilitation services for persons with
> multiple sclerosis in Europe
>
> 1. Provision of appropriate respite care and short breaks for both
>   the carer and the person with MS
> 2. Provision of appropriate long-term facilities
> 3. Access to information about services and community care
>   resources
> 4. Expertise in caring for persons with MS with severe disability
> 5. Coordination of all services
> 6. Adequate and appropriate community care services, including
>   home adaptations, mobility equipment and aids, health
>   services
> 7. Appropriate palliative care

Charles' experience

The physio- and occupational therapists were inspiring and
highly effective. They identified my deteriorating condition,
persuaded me of its seriousness and identified an appropriate course of therapy. They also designed proper support
from my wheel-chair, all with infectious enthusiasm and
charm. I cannot speak too highly of them.

Poor selection of a device can impact on symptoms, complicate
a person's life and hinder everyday activities. The base, and each
component of the chair such as support surface, key seating
angle, upholstery, height, width and foot and armrests must be
considered.[64] In addition, broader and longer-term issues in
device choice, such as repairs, guarantees, transportability and
esthetics are important factors. MS healthcare professionals
should be aware of the key factors that should be considered in
the assessment for and recommendation of wheeled mobility aids
(Box 2.11).[64]

Resource implications

As a complex, unpredictable condition MS does not fit easily into
healthcare structures. As knowledge of MS pathology expands
and diagnostic interventions and therapeutic treatments develop,

Box 2.11. Assessment for and recommendation of wheeled mobility aids (adapted from reference 64)

- Recognize the complexity of selecting a wheeled mobility device for a person with MS
- Recognize the need for a comprehensive and skilled assessment by seating and mobility specialists (usually occupational therapists and physiotherapists) to work with the person with MS to select the most appropriate device
- Identify factors related to the individual, the device, the environment and lifestyle issues that need to be considered in the selection process
- Teach people with MS which questions to ask when purchasing wheeled mobility devices

a larger population of people with MS will become eligible for treatment, increasing healthcare costs. One of the most controversial areas of MS care is the allocation of financial resources to disease-modifying drug treatment budgets. The objective of disease-modifying drug therapies is to temporarily reduce disability due to relapses. There has been debate about the use of costly disease-modifying drugs which have an impact on relapses but have scarce and controversial data on effect on disease progression.

As with all long-term conditions the potential for short-term cost offsets is limited, as the major cost drivers are dependence due to physical disability and the loss of work due to worsening disease. To date it has been difficult to ascertain the true economic cost of MS due to variation in data collection systems and models used. It is now recognized that there is a need to create an integrated model that represents the disease in a structured way estimating the cost effectiveness of treatments from medium- to long-term or lifetime periods.[65]

Whilst debates regarding economic models of MS care take place, the need for people with MS to be supported to access timely appropriate specialist services prevails. It is the role of MS healthcare professionals to minimize impact of this disease by delivering evidence-based, quality care. MS rehabilitation teams may need to compete for and harness resources in order to deliver a quality service in the most appropriate environment.

Charles' experience of inpatient rehabilitation

The three weeks in seclusion gave me an invaluable opportunity for self-analysis and self-appraisal at an important stage in my life. The benefits stay with me.

Other aspects of the three weeks were of less relevance to me with my form of primary progressive MS. I did not have many medical needs; nursing staff offered some useful advice on some catheterization and continence. It is difficult to see, however, how a residential rehabilitation unit sited in a hospital can be the best way of preparing people for independent living. The physical layout of the bathrooms, for instance, bore no resemblance to anything in private accommodation and no disabled person could have been involved in the positioning of a bath, free standing in the middle of a room without anywhere for soap, towels or support.

To me the hospital culture stifled the rehabilitation; hospital beds, hospital food, hospital hours, central dispensing of drugs. I sound ungrateful but for me there must be more efficient ways of dispensing twelve hours of invaluable therapy.

Most of my fellow patients were of the relapsing–remitting form and I am in the minority; nevertheless all of us have lived with MS, some of us for many years, and little or no use was made of our expertise and experience of independent living. The other frustration is the lack of subsequent support on returning home. Once home, subsequent close liaison with local services is vital. In my view any course of rehabilitation aimed at returning people home cannot be based in a hospital.

The fundamental principles of quality MS services which should underpin any model of MS service have been summarized by the European Multiple Sclerosis Platform[63] (Box 2.12), components of a quality service (Box 2.13) and key themes for teamwork and service delivery (Box 2.14).

Summary

MS is a long-term condition which has an enormous impact on a person's life. Health and social care professionals should endeavor

Box 2.12. Important qualities to underpin MS service delivery.[63] Recommendations on rehabilitation services for persons with multiple sclerosis in Europe

- The service must guarantee internal integration among professionals and must also be integrated with all other existing health services relevant for MS (hospital departments, outpatient clinics, community services), so that gaps in service delivery and communication are avoided
- Because MS is unpredictable, particularly with regard to relapse occurrence and speed of disability progression, response should be in a timely manner without excessive delay or bureaucracy
- There is a variety of symptoms, disabilities and disease subtypes; services must be flexible and able to adapt to the needs of patients
- Services should be patient centered, available to all patients, and not designed to meet the institution or funder's needs; services must be as close in proximity to the patients as resources allow
- Services must be evidence based. This encompasses practicing evidence-based care but also draws from relevant research in non-MS areas and collaborates to build the evidence base through research and audit

Box 2.13. Resource and capacity considerations.[63] Recommendations on rehabilitation services for persons with multiple sclerosis in Europe

- Adherence to fundamental principles means that funding must be available for appropriate integration of services, as a person with MS may access inpatient, outpatient and community services to different degrees at different stages of the illness
- In order to be patient centered and provide timely services, there must be some uncommitted capacity to treating urgent, unforeseen needs, such as relapses or an atypical disease course
- A good MS service will not allocate all clinical resources to planned patients as it recognizes the need for flexibility. In order to improve current and future care, all services need time and support to contribute to research and audit

Box 2.14. Key themes for teamwork and service delivery in MS.[63] Recommendations on rehabilitation services for persons with multiple sclerosis in Europe

- Rehabilitation is a process, a continuum, provided by a highly trained and informed team
- Teamwork is dynamic and flexible, tailored according to the needs of the person with MS
- On the basis of thorough assessment, the team should set achievable goals that can be measured
- Team work with the person with MS should be interdisciplinary, needs to share common stable values but retain openness to change
- The person with MS and his/her carer are key members of the team
- The team has core members whose input is necessary more frequently during the course of MS
- Delivered services should be of high quality but as accessible as possible (home based if feasible)
- Delivery of services should be continuously adapted to the needs of the person with MS and should be flexible, timely, evidence and experienced based
- Delivery of services for the person with MS and their carers should be accessible and regionally equal (home based if the quality is sustained)

to support individuals so that they can make appropriate adaptations and maximize self-management strategies. Professionals have much to learn from people with MS and should find ways to encourage their involvement, sharing platforms so that their voices can be heard. It is only when professionals and people with MS join forces to share experience/knowledge to work together that truly user-focused services will be designed and delivered. Appropriate, timely, quality-based services could go a long way to minimize the impact of this disease.

Ben

I feel confident about the future, knowing that I have a rock of support at the specialist center and also that I am doing all that I can for myself in terms of diet, exercise and overall lifestyle. I've taken on board all advice I've been given, in particular with regard to diet, and exercise, and making life as simple as possible. I lead a well-managed life, and I strive for no surprises and I feel fully prepared for whatever challenges lie ahead.

References

1. Rieckmann P (2004) Improving MS care. J Neurol 251: 69–73.
2. Mohr DC, Dick LP, Russo D et al (1999) The psychosocial impact of multiple sclerosis: exploring the patient's perspective. Health Psychol 18: 376–82.
3. Holman HR, Lorig K (2000) Patients as partners in managing chronic disease. BMJ 320: 526–7.
4. Department of Health (2001) The expert patient: a new approach to chronic disease management for the 21st century. London, HMSO.
5. Lorig KR, Holman H (2003) Self-management education: history, definition, outcomes, and mechanisms. Ann Behav Med 26: 1–7.
6. Murray TJ (1995) The psychosocial aspects of multiple sclerosis. Neurol Clin 13: 197–223.
7. Somerset M, Campbell R, Sharp DJ, Peters TJ (2001) What do people with MS want and expect from MS services? Health Expect 4: 29–37.
8. Department of Health (2005) Improving chronic disease management. London, Department of Health.
9. Koopman W, Schweitzer A (1999) The journey to multiple sclerosis: a qualitative study. J Neurosci Nurs 31: 17–26.
10. Robinson I (1991) The context and consequences of communicating the diagnosis of multiple sclerosis: some brief findings from a survey of 900 patients. In: Wietholder H, Dickgans J, Merten J, eds. Current Concepts in Multiple Sclerosis. New York, Elsevier: 17–22.
11. Robinson I (1996) The Views of People with MS About their Needs. Birmingham, Brunel Research Unit.
12. Wollin J, Dale H, Spenser N, Walsh A (2000) What people with newly diagnosed MS (and their families and friends need to know). Int J MS Care 2: 3–4.
13. Freeman J, Johnson J, Rollinson S et al. (1997) Standards of Healthcare for People with Multiple Sclerosis. London, Multiple Sclerosis Society of Great Britain and Northern Ireland and The National Hospital for Neurology and Neurosurgery.
14. Halper J (1999) The needs of people who are newly diagnosed with multiple sclerosis. MS Management 1–4
15. Stewart MA (1995) Effective physician–patient communication and health outcomes: a review. Can Med Assoc J 152: 1423–33.

16. Coulter A (2001) Quality of hospital care: measuring patients' experiences. Proc R Coll Physicians Edinb 31(Suppl 9): 34–6.

17. Leary S, Porter B, Thompson A (2005) Multiple sclerosis: diagnosis and the management of acute relapses. Postgrad Med J 81: 302–8.

18. McDonald WI, Compston A, Edan G, et al. (2001) Recommended diagnostic criteria for multiple sclerosis: guidelines from the international panel on the diagnosis of multiple sclerosis. Ann Neurol 50: 121–7.

19. Craig J, Young CA, Ennis M, et al. (2003) A randomised controlled trial comparing rehabilitation against standard therapy in multiple sclerosis patients receiving intravenous steroid treatment. J Neurol Neurosurg Psychiatry 74: 1225–30.

20. Liu C, Playford ED, Thompson AJ (2003) Does neurorehabilitation have a role in relapsing–remitting multiple sclerosis. J Neurol 250: 1214–18.

21. National Institute for Clinical Excellence (2003) Management of Multiple Sclerosis in Primary and Secondary Care. London, NICE.

22. Multiple Sclerosis Society UK (2005) MS Essentials II Diet and Nutrition. MS105.

23. Bakshi R, Shaikh ZA, Miletech RS et al. (2000) Fatigue in multiple sclerosis and its relationship to depression and neurological disability. Mult Scler 6: 181–5.

24. Herbert I, Karpatkin PT (2005) Multiple sclerosis and exercise: a review of the evidence. Int J MS Care 7: 36–41.

25. Petajan JH, Gappmaier E, White AT et al. (1996) Impact on aerobic training on fitness and quality of life in multiple sclerosis. Ann Neurol 39: 432–41.

26. Harvey L, Smith AD, Jones R (1999) The effect of weighted leg raises on quadriceps strength, EMG parameters, and functional activities in people with multiple sclerosis. Physiotherapy 85: 154–61.

27. Smeltzer SC, Lavietes MH, Cook SD (1996) Expiratory training in multiple sclerosis. Arch Phys Med Rehabil 77: 909–12.

28. Rumill P (2006) Help to stay at work: vocational rehabilitation. MS Focus 7: 14–15.

29. O'Connor RJ, Thompson AJ, Playford ED (2005) Does the clinician have a role in work retention for people with multiple sclerosis? Cross-sectional studies using qualitative and quantitative methods. J Neurol 8: 892–6.

30. Larocca N, Kalb R, Kendall P, Scheinberg L (1982) The role of disease and demographic factors in the employment of patients with multiple sclerosis. Arch Neurol 39: 256.

31. Gronning M, Hannisdal E, Mellgren SI (1990) Multivariate analyses of factors associated with unemployment in people with multiple sclerosis. J Neurol Neurosurg Psychiatry 53: 388–90.

32. Department of Health (2005) The National Service Framework for Long term Conditions. London, Department of Health.

33. www.direct.gov.uk

34. Confareux C, Hutchinson M, Hours MM et al. (1998) Rate of pregnancy-related relapse in multiple sclerosis. Pregnancy in Multiple Sclerosis Group. N Engl J Med 339: 285–91.

35. Bennett KA (2005) Pregnancy and multiple sclerosis. Clin Obstet Gynaecol 48: 38–47.

36. Neild C (2005) Sex, intimacy and relationships. MS Essentials. UK MS Society 12.

37. Kalb R (2004) What is it about MS that makes it a family disease? MS Focus 3: 4–5.

38. Nabe-Nielsen M (2004) How to encourage your children to talk about MS. MS Focus 3: 6–8.

39. Schrag A, Morley D, Quinn N, Jahanshahi M (2004) Development of a measure of the impact of chronic parental illness on adolescent and adult children: The Impact of Parental Illness Questionnaire (Parkinson's Disease). Parkinsonism and Related Disorders, 10: 399–405.

40. Mutch K (2005) Information for young people when multiple sclerosis enters the family. Br J Nurs 14: 758–60.

41. Pollizi C, Plamisano L, Mainero C et al. (2004) Relationship between emotional distress in caregivers and health status in persons with multiple sclerosis. Mult Scler 10: 442–6.

42. Aronson KJ (1997) Quality of life among persons with multiple sclerosis and their caregivers. Neurology 48: 74–80.

43. Dewis MME, Niskala H (1992) Nurturing a valuable resource: family care givers in multiple sclerosis. Axon 13: 87–94.

44. Sato A, Ricks K, Watkins S (1996) Needs of caregivers of clients with multiple sclerosis. J Commun Health Nurs 13: 31–42.

45. Wollin J, Reiher C, Spencer N, Madl R, Nutter H (1999) Caregiver burden: meeting the needs of people who support the person with multiple sclerosis. Int J MS Care 2: 6–15.

46. Weinert C, Long KA (1993) Support systems for the spouses of chronically ill persons in rural areas. Fam Commun Health 16: 46–54.

47. Good DM, Bower DA, Einsporn RL (1995) Social support: gender differences in multiple sclerosis spousal caregivers. J Neurosci Nurs 27: 305–11.

48. Winslow B, O' Brien R (1992) Use of formal community resources by spouse caregivers of chronically ill adults. Public Health Nurs 9: 128–32.

49. Aronson KL, Cleghorn G, Goldenberg E (1996) Assistance arrangements and use of services among persons with multiple sclerosis and their caregivers. Disabil Rehabil 18: 354–61.

50. Springer RA, Clark S, Price E, Weldon P (2001) Psychosocial implications of multiple sclerosis. In: Advanced Concepts in Multiple Sclerosis Nursing Care. New York, Demos: 213–37.

51. Strittamer R (2004) Emotion-related issues of the newly diagnosed. MS Focus 4: 7–9.
52. Sadovnick AD, Remick RA, Allen J et al. (1996) Depression and multiple sclerosis. Neurology 46: 628–32.
53. Rost K, Zhang M, Fortney J et al. (1998) Persistently poor outcomes of undetected major depression in primary care. Gen Hosp Psychiatry 20: 12–20.
54. Perez-Stable E, Miranda J, Munoz R, Ying YW (1990) Depression in medical outpatients: under recognition and misdiagnosis. Arch Intern Med 150: 1083–8
55. Badger L, deGruy F, Hartman J et al. (1994) Patient presentation, interview content and the detection of depression in primary care physicians. Psychosom Med 56: 128–35.
56. Feinstein A (1997) Multiple sclerosis, depression and suicide. BMJ 315: 691–2.
57. Stenager EN, Stenager E, Koch-Herikson N et al. (1992) Suicide and multiple sclerosis: an epidemiological investigation. J Neurol Neurosurg Psychiatry 55: 542–5.
58. Zoron M, De Masi R, Nausuelli D et al. (2001) Depression and anxiety in multiple sclerosis: a clinical and MRI study in 95 subjects. J Neurol 248: 416–21.
59. La Rocca N (2004) Introducing MS-related emotional and cognitive issues. MS Focus 4: 4–6.
60. Cockerill R, Warren S (1990) Care for caregivers: the needs of family members of MS patients. J Rehabil 56: 41–4.
61. De Rosier MB, Cantanzaro M, Piller J (1992) Living with chronic illness: social support and the well spouse perspective. Rehabil Nurse 17: 87–91.
62. Kalb R (2003) Multiple sclerosis a model for psychosocial support. New York, National Multiple Sclerosis Society.
63. European Multiple Sclerosis Platform (2004) Recommendations on rehabilitation services for persons with multiple sclerosis in Europe.
64. Finlayson M, Winter R (2003) Wheeled mobility – evidence and expertise. Int J MS Care 7: 85–6.
65. Kobelt G (2006) Health economic issues in MS. Int MS J 13: 16–26.

3

Multidisciplinary rehabilitation

E Diane Playford

While current evidence supports the provision of well organized, co-ordinated, multidisciplinary rehabilitation services based on a problem-oriented approach in stroke,[1] and traumatic brain injury,[2] the evidence base for multiple sclerosis (MS) and other progressive neurological conditions is weaker. Welcome advances include a refining of the concepts that underpin rehabilitation, increasing numbers of studies evaluating aspects of neurological rehabilitation and increasing sophistication in measuring outcomes.

Effective management of MS demands an awareness of the impact of the disease as it progresses, and the development of systems that allow the appropriate referral of an individual with MS between different services and disciplines. Key to delivering comprehensive and joined-up care is a shared understanding and language when describing disability and its management.

Rehabilitation concepts

The international classification of impairments, disabilities, and handicaps (ICIDH) was developed under the auspices of the World Health Organization and was first published in 1980.[3] The ICIDH has recently been revised and is now known as the International Classification of Functioning, Disability and Health (ICF).[4] The overall aim of the ICF classification is to provide a unified and standard language and framework for the description of health and health-related states. The ICF classifies functioning at the levels of body/body part, whole person and whole person in social context. Disablements are:

1. Losses or abnormalities of bodily function and structure (impairments)
2. Limitations of activities (formerly disabilities)
3. Restrictions in participation (formerly called handicaps)

Functioning is therefore an umbrella term encompassing all body functions, activities and participation; similarly, disability serves as an umbrella term for impairments, activity limitations or participation restrictions. Box 3.1 shows that disablement and functioning are outcomes of interactions between health conditions and personal and contextual factors. Two sorts of contextual factors are identified: social and physical environmental factors (social attitudes, access to buildings, legal protection etc.); and personal factors that include gender, age, other health conditions, social background, education, overall behavior pattern and other factors that influence how disablement is experienced by the individual.

Box 3.1. International classification of function

The definitions of the levels of functioning in the ICF in the context of a Health Condition...

Impairment is a loss or abnormality of body structure or of a physiological or psychological function, e.g. loss of a limb, loss of vision...

Activity is the nature and extent of functioning at the level of the person. Activities may be limited in nature, duration and quality, e.g. taking care of oneself, maintaining a job...

Participation is the nature and extent of a person's involvement in life situations in relation to Impairment, Activities, Health Conditions and Contextual Factors. Participation may be restricted in nature, duration and quality, e.g. participation in community activities, obtaining a driving licence...

Multidisciplinary rehabilitation therefore focuses on managing the impact of MS on an individual's activity and participation in the context of both environmental and personal factors. There are a number of different definitions of rehabilitation[5–7] (Box 3.2) but current thinking would place the individual with MS at the center of the process, making them an integral member of the team, so that they acquire the knowledge, skills, attitudes and support they need to ameliorate those aspects of the impact of MS that they regard as important. Thus, the aims of rehabilitation will vary between individuals. In general the aim is for an individual and their families to be able to maintain their autonomy, and maximize the level of activity and participation. This includes the prevention of complications and secondary disability.

Much is written about different models of rehabilitation but the features of a successful specialist rehabilitation team are probably similar to those of expert teams in other fields such as stroke or diabetes management. The British Society of Rehabilitation Medicine has recently proposed clinical standards for inpatient specialist rehabilitation services in the UK.[8] These standards relate to both the structures and the processes by which rehabilitation is delivered.

Box 3.2. Definitions of rehabilitation

A process of active change by which a person who has become disabled acquires the knowledge and skills needed for optimum physical, psychological and social functioning[5]

The application of all measures aimed at reducing the impact of disabling and handicapping conditions, and enabling disabled and handicapped people to achieve social integration[5]

The process of restoration to the maximum degree possible of function (physical or mental) or role (within the family, social network, or workforce)[6]

A problem-solving and educational process aimed at reducing the disability and handicap experienced by someone as a result of disease, always within the limitations imposed both by available resources and by the underlying disease[7]

Structure

The multidisciplinary team

The concept of a multidisciplinary team is central to a rehabilitation service. Common core team members include specialists in nursing, physiotherapy and occupational therapy. Access to speech and language therapists, dietetics, orthotics, wheelchair services, environmental control services, psychology and counseling services and social workers are also helpful.[8] Specialist neurological rehabilitation teams include a neurologist or rehabilitation physician who is skilled in the management of neurological disability, in addition to the other members of the multidisciplinary team. The role of the physician is to provide an accurate diagnosis, prognostic information and advice about symptomatic management.

The team needs to have a geographical base, meet regularly and have adequate administrative support.[8] For the team to function well, they should have a clearly defined remit, and work with the individual with MS to formulate multidisciplinary goals in addition to unidisciplinary goals. Relatively little research has been done into the functioning of multidisciplinary teams in medicine, but problems may arise due to the interpersonal skills or when the unidisciplinary aims of an individual discipline conflict with the aims of the team. Individuals need to feel confident in their ability to delegate tasks within the team.

Principles of therapy

All of the disciplines described below have a number of principles in common. One principle that is common to them all is that the therapy should be patient-centered and tailored to the patient's specific needs and ambitions. Another is that patients can be empowered by education and thus enabled to continue the therapeutic process after the intervention by the therapist has been completed. A third is that prevention is better than cure; thus most therapists believe that they should see people with MS early to provide education about the approaches to preventing avoidable complications such as poor posture, tone management difficulties, contractures, frequent falls and incontinence which can impact on social roles such as employment.

The role of the MS nurse

An MS nurse is an experienced health care professional with specific training in MS who can provide expert help and advice for people with MS and their carers regarding:[9]

- New symptoms
- Coping with diagnosis/disability
- Advice on local resources
- Treatment options and availability
- Information about the disease

MS specialist nurses differ in a number of ways and the precise nature of their role will depend on whether they are in a neurology clinic, a rehabilitation unit or working in the community. Whatever the setting, their key role will include assessment and management of MS symptoms and the co-ordination of care, helping individuals, where possible, reach their goals of self-management.

The role of the rehabilitation nurse

The contribution of the rehabilitation nurse is crucial to successful inpatient rehabilitation. It differs from the traditional nursing role of providing care to one of facilitation of independence, allowing the carryover of new skills learnt with the therapists to the more day-to-day environment of the ward.[10] In addition nurses develop specific areas of expertise including bladder and bowel management, skin care and the management of pressure sores, counseling and education about specific conditions.

The role of the occupational therapist

Occupational therapists[11] enable people to achieve health, wellbeing, independence and life satisfaction through participation in occupation: that is, the daily activities that an individual undertakes and which define identify and provide self-esteem.[12] Occupation may be considered under three key areas: productivity (work), leisure and self-care. Thus occupational therapists will work with people with MS to help them to participate, at whatever level they are able, in these areas in a way that the person with MS considers to be most meaningful and relevant.

Occupational therapists utilize their specialist skills to solve practical problems, such as fatigue, by

- Working with the individual to learn or re-learn ways in which activities can be successfully carried out, through specific treatment techniques
- Adapting the activity itself, for example by advising on specialist equipment to assist in carrying it out, or learning a new technique
- Modifying the environment in which an activity is carried out, for example by changing attitudes/the environment within the workplace, or designing housing adaptations to remove or minimize obstacles
- Educating and advising individuals on alternative occupations or activities in the context of their difficulties

The role of the speech and language therapist

People affected by MS may present with a variety of speech, language and swallowing symptoms.[13] The speech and language therapist[11] will assess the pattern of communication and swallowing problems and, in consultation with the person affected by MS, determine the most effective way to manage these. Typical interventions include working with individuals to maintain clarity of speech, providing appropriate augmentative and alternative communication devices, and working to support effective interaction and communication skills, enabling the individual to participate in conversation and decision-making processes. For patients with swallowing difficulties speech therapists will assess the swallow and then advise on techniques that promote safe and effective swallowing and, where appropriate, provide advice about supplementary feeding.

The role of the physiotherapist

Physiotherapy is a physical and educational treatment approach which is concerned with maximizing mobility, movement and function.[11] The primary aims of physiotherapy are to restore and maintain function, activity and independence and to prevent injury or illness through treatment, information and advice on healthy lifestyles.[14]

Physiotherapists will work with patients at all stages of their MS. Early after diagnosis they have an important educational role encouraging and motivating individuals to maintain cardiovascular fitness and overall health and wellbeing through specialist treatment and exercise programs. Subsequently they have important roles in helping individuals

- Learn self-management techniques
- Improve and/or maintain muscle activity, balance, mobility, posture and joint range
- Develop strategies to manage symptoms such as pain and spasticity
- Maintain their independent and safe functional ability

The role of a key worker

Many patients undergoing rehabilitation have complex neurological disability requiring input from a number of different disciplines often based in geographically distinct locations. For example, at the point of discharge, a single patient may have links with six different disciplines in hospital, a hospital-based outpatient physiotherapy service, community-based occupational therapy, a social worker and carers employed by social services and a local housing department. Co-ordination of all these workers is crucial to the success of the discharge and the maintenance of functional status. A key worker's role is to co-ordinate these services and provide a single point of contact for the patient and family.[15]

Process

Rehabilitation as a process has a number of discrete elements, including assessment, goal setting, treatment and evaluation.[16]

Assessment

The quality of the intervention will depend on the accuracy of the analysis of the presenting problems. Many patients have complex interacting problems, and defining the contribution of each element to a particular problem is essential before embarking on treatment whether therapy or pharmaceutically based. Assessment therefore involves identifying the most productive focus for interventions, the order in which they should occur and the environment in which they should take place.

A number of different approaches to assessment may be used, but most depend on the input of a multidisciplinary team to define impairment, and identify activity and participation issues. Different disciplines have particular skills at identifying particular disabilities; for example, being at risk of pressure sores is clearly identified by nurses but poorly identified by other team members.[17]

This expert assessment results in identification of a series of potential outcomes. The next step is to identify those which are priorities for the individual with MS. Having agreed on an overall aim, it is common practice for the individual and the team to devise a workable strategy consisting of a sequence of pragmatic achievable goals, to achieve the desired aim. This process of negotiating goals is widely referred to as 'goal setting'.

Goal setting

Goal setting refers to a process of discussion and negotiation in which the individual with MS and the multidisciplinary team determine the key priorities for rehabilitation for that individual, and agree the performance level to be attained by the patient for defined activities within a specified time frame.

The language used to describe goals varies from center to center, but typically many services will articulate a long-term goal that has a time frame of months, and short-term goals which define the steps needed to accomplish the long-term goal.

The theoretical basis for goal setting in rehabilitation derives from two sources: the psychology literature and the rehabilitation literature. The main source is the vast organizational psychology literature published in the 1970s investigating the effectiveness of goal setting in improving productivity within the workplace.

Recently, Locke and Latham (2002) synthesized the results from a number of studies exploring the effectiveness of goal setting from the literature, with a total involvement of 40 000 participants.[18] The results demonstrate increased goal-orientated performance on over 100 different tasks based across eight countries in field, laboratory and simulated settings. Studies demonstrate that goal setting improves productivity and performance in a wide range of occupations,[19–22] sports[23,24] and education.[25,26]

There are three key findings of these studies:

- Challenging goals lead to better performance[27–29]
- Participative goals tend to be more demanding than assigned goals[30–32]
- Goal setting is more effective when goals are specific.[29,33] The goal should be clearly defined in terms of both purpose and duration

It is from these studies that the concept of SMART goals has been developed – i.e. that goals need to be specific, measurable, achievable, relevant and time limited.[34] While the findings from these studies have been adopted in rehabilitation practice, these psychology studies presented goals that were often simple and constrained, and were performed within an experimental paradigm. Rehabilitation is concerned with complex issues in a changing environment and, in the case of MS, may be complicated by accruing disability.

There are now a growing number of clinical studies of goal setting, although none specifically in MS.[35] Typically these studies have examined people with brain injury, or the elderly. One important finding is that cognitive impairment may be no barrier to individuals setting realistic and achievable goals.[36,37] As demonstrated in the psychology literature there is evidence that both challenging goals[37] and participative goals result in better outcomes.[38]

In summary, goal setting is a technique used to determine the key priorities for an the rehabilitation of an individual. There are clear reasons for involving the individual with MS in goal setting and setting demanding goals. Once goals have been set, the multidisciplinary team can start to work with the individual to achieve those goals.

Treatment

Goal setting initiates a treatment program. The changes that occur in the patient's condition as a result of the treatment program needs to be monitored and the treatment program revised appropriately. Treatment uses all available means to achieve a desired outcome. This may include medical treatments, surgical interventions, therapy-based treatments or the provision of different forms of support and care. Following a successful outcome the process may be repeated or an active decision made to discontinue at this stage. Often a number of different problems are identified and patients will be at different stages of the process for each problem. For this reason it is essential to have regular review periods in which the benefits can be evaluated and the reasons for failure to make progress can be identified.

Evaluation

Rehabilitation is an iterative process. After treatment the impact of the intervention should be evaluated, and then any remaining problems assessed and, if necessary, treated. Evaluation may be performed in a number of different ways. This includes document-ing the compliance with a defined care pathway, recording goal achievement or the use of standardized outcome measures.

The evaluation of process is facilitated by the development of an integrated care pathway (ICP). An ICP consists of a document which maps the interventions that should occur during a specific episode of patient care.[39] It allows evidence-based guidelines to be embedded into local practice. Developing them is an intera-tive process and should represent consensus about best practice. Rehabilitation ICPs consist of three elements – the pathway, the goal categories sheet and the variance sheet.[40]

The benefits of ICPs lie in specifying the best possible method of delivering care and in describing the patterns of variances. A variance sheet may be used to record either departures from the pathway (procedural variance) or the reasons for non-achieve-ment of goals. Individual variances are neither good nor bad. They are simply a method of recording what happened to a specific patient and the reasons for it, thus allowing for individ-ualized patient care. The patterns of variances across a group of patients will identify strengths and weaknesses in the processes around particular episodes of care and permit incorporation of new ideas and remediation of problems. When combined with measurement tools it is possible to identify which aspects of care impact positively or adversely on the outcome.

Goals may be categorized and analyzed to ensure that the full range of disabilities and handicaps are being covered, and to identify areas of weakness and strength in treatment programs.[41]

Once embedded in the clinical processes, data collection using ICPs becomes routine but regular analysis of the pathway and subsequent modification of the pathway and associated variance codes requires continuing commitment and support from a speci-fied staff member.

The evaluation of outcome is equally important. Most units now routinely incorporate standardized outcome measures into patient assessment at admission and discharge. There are now a wide variety of measures available; the selection of an appropri-ate measure depends on the clinical setting and the anticipated effect of the intervention. The advantages of using outcome measures routinely are that they permit comparison between one unit and another, and allow the grouping of patients into differ-ent bands for inclusion in clinical trials (see Chapter 5).

Stages of MS

MS is characterized by changing patterns of need.[42] In order to provide a framework within which the needs of an individual can be accurately identified and met, it is helpful to consider four separate stages in the evolution of the disease: diagnosis; minimal disability; moderate disability; and severe disability.[43] The boundaries between these stages may be poorly defined but the management of relapses may be encompassed within the 'minimal disability' stage, moderate disability requires both symptomatic management and rehabilitation, whereas severe disability additionally demands co-ordinated delivery of care in the community, and an awareness of end-of-life issues. Patient education and self-management, core rehabilitation concepts, underpin the management at all stages of the disease.

Minimal disability

In the treatment of minimal disability, the main focus is on self-management with an emphasis on the concept of wellness incorporating diet, exercise and a healthy lifestyle. Stuifbergen and colleagues conducted a study of 112 women for a total of 8 months using a two-phase intervention program including lifestyle-change classes for 8 weeks.[44] The follow-up suggested an increase in self-efficacy for health behaviors, health-promoting behaviors, and the mental health and pain scales of the SF-36. Maintaining a good diet may be of particular importance and particular difficulty for people with increasing disability. A recent review[45] emphasized the importance of nutrition in MS and the evidence underpinning dietary advice.

A recent Cochrane review assessed the effectiveness of exercise therapy for patients with MS in terms of activities of daily living and health-related quality of life.[46] Synthesis of six high-quality randomized controlled trials involving 164 participants compared one or two exercise therapy interventions with a no-treatment condition.[47–52] The synthesis suggested that there is strong evidence in favor of exercise therapy compared to no-exercise therapy in terms of muscle power function, exercise tolerance functions and mobility-related activities. Moderate evidence was found for improving mood. No evidence was observed for exercise therapy on fatigue and perception of handicap when compared to no-exercise therapy. The results suggest that exercise therapy, whether similar to that recommended for the healthy population or modified to simply maintain function, does have efficacy in MS.

One issue of importance at this stage of the disease is the management of relapses. The use of steroids is well established, and the NICE guidelines suggest that any individual who experiences an acute episode (including optic neuritis) sufficient to cause distressing symptoms or an increased limitation on activities should be offered a course of high-dose corticosteroids.[53] The course should be started as soon as possible after onset of the relapse and should be either intravenous methylprednisolone (IVMP) 500 mg–1 g daily, for between 3 and 5 days or high-dose oral methylprednisolone 500 mg–2 g daily, for between 3 and 5 days. However, the individual should understand the risks and benefits involved in using steroids and frequent (more than three times a year) or prolonged (longer than 3 weeks) use of corticosteroids should be avoided. Intravenous steroids may be given either at home or in a hospital setting. There is little evidence to support either setting. Potential benefits of home administration include patient preference, decreased infection risk, and lower indirect costs, particularly in terms of patient's and carer time lost from work. A recent study suggested that people with MS prefer home administration and that there is no difference in costs between home and hospital intervention.[54]

A further issue to consider is the role of multidisciplinary rehabilitation following a relapse. Up to 40% of relapses may leave some residual problems,[55] and there is evidence that improvement of impairments and disability after treatment with IVMP for a relapse of MS occurs early, while improvement of subjective health status is delayed.[56] A recent randomized controlled trial evaluated the benefits of IVMP with planned, comprehensive, multidisciplinary team care compared with IVMP with standard care. The control group (20 patients) was managed according to the standard ward routine; the treatment group (20 patients) received planned co-ordinated multidisciplinary team assessment and treatment. Results showed statistically significant differences in Guys Neurological Disability Scale and the Barthel Index (BI) ($p = 0.02$) at 3 months in favor of planned multidisciplinary care.[57] This finding was supported by audit data from a neurorehabilitation service that demonstrated that individuals with relapsing–remitting MS showed considerable improvement following rehabilitation, with a median change of –0.5 on Expanded Disability Status Scale (EDSS), +4 on BI and +12 on Functional Impact Measure (FIM). Patients valued their admissions with their perceived benefit correlating with improvements in disability measures.[58]

Moderate disability

Two randomized studies were published at the end of the 1990s which suggested that rehabilitation was of benefit to people with moderate disability due to MS. Freeman and colleagues[59] reported on 66 patients with progressive MS using a wait-list controlled study and demonstrated that short periods of inpatient rehabilitation resulted in improvements in both disability and handicap compared with those in the wait-list control group.[59] A follow-up study demonstrated that the gains made were sustained for up to 6 months.[60] These key findings were supported by Solari and colleagues who studied 50 patients randomly assigned to a home exercise program or inpatient rehabilitation. At the end of the intervention the study group improved significantly in disability and the improvement had persisted at 9 weeks.[61]

More recently studies have demonstrated the benefit of outpatient rehabilitation.[62,63] The benefits of multidisciplinary rehabilitation have been demonstrated usually through improvements in measures of disability, handicap and quality of life, whilst impairment remains unchanged. It remains unclear, however, which elements of the rehabilitation package are effective.

There are a small number of studies of individual therapy disciplines. Two studies report on physiotherapy. Lord and colleagues (1998) compared two physiotherapy approaches (impairment vs. disability based, ten patients in each group) both of which resulted in improvements in mobility as measured using the 10-meter timed walk, the Rivermead Mobility Index, stride length and the Rivermead Visual Gait Assessment.[64] Balance was assessed using the Berg Balance Test. Wiles and colleagues[52] performed a randomized controlled crossover trial in patients with chronic MS who had difficulty walking. Allocation was to one of six permutations of three 8-week treatment periods separated by 8-week intervals: treatments consisted of physiotherapy at home, as an outpatient, or 'no therapy'. On the

Rivermead Mobility Index (scale 0–15) (primary outcome) there was a highly significant (p <0.001) treatment effect of 1.4–1.5 units favoring hospital or home-based therapy over no therapy. This was supported by other measures of mobility, gait, balance and the assessor's global 'mobility change' score: there was no major difference between home and hospital.

A recent Cochrane review of the role of occupational therapy in MS aimed to determine whether occupational therapy interventions in MS patients improved functional ability, social participation and/or health-related quality of life.[65] There was a lack of well-designed studies in the area. Lack of evidence does not, of course, equate to lack of efficacy, but does highlight the need for well-designed studies in the future. Such studies ideally need to follow the Medical Research Council (MRC) guidance on the evaluation of complex interventions.[66]

Severe disability

Once an individual becomes more severely disabled, access to hospital-based services becomes more difficult and the importance of both formal and informal care networks increases. Management tends to be based within the community. The aims of management remain similar, focusing on maintaining autonomy, supporting the individual and their carers in decision making, providing information and ensuring co-ordination of care.

Recent work has focused on the role of palliative care in people with long-term conditions. The importance of palliative care approaches has recently been highlighted by the National Service Framework for Long Term (Neurological) Conditions, in which quality requirement 9 addresses the need for palliative care services for people in the advanced stages of neurological conditions and the importance of enabling people to make choices about end-of-life care.[67] A recent paper highlights the emotional and physical difficulties faced by people with MS including disbelief and devastation; losses and forced life choices; tracking down services and information; and sadness and relief.[68] The NICE guidance for supportive and palliative care for adults with cancer sets out the benchmark for palliative care services.[69] While these principles were developed within cancer services the recommendations apply to end-of-life care in all conditions. Discussing end-of-life issues and preparing an advance directive help allay anxiety and fear. Many of the symptoms experienced in the advanced stages of MS may be similar to those in cancer[70] (e.g. in terms of pain and breathlessness[71]), but some aspects of management may differ. For example, managing pain arising from spasticity or neuropathic pain needs a different approach from managing cancer pain (see Chapter 4). Cognitive and communication problems may impact on an individual's ability to understand complex information, describe their symptoms, make choices, and express their concerns and desires around end-of-life issues clearly. Professionals may need support in helping to provide information appropriately.\

Although conceptually it may be easier to conceive of individuals with MS as passing through four distinct phases, in reality this is simply an approach to organizing service. Some individuals may want to discuss end-of-life issues at diagnosis, others with high levels of dependency may need information about diagnosis. However, key themes underpin the management of MS at all stages of the disease. As with all individuals, people with MS and their families want to be autonomous individuals able to decide the best management for themselves. To enable this, services must provide appropriate information tailored to the individual's needs and responsive, co-ordinated and expert services. \

References

1. Stroke Unit Trialists' Collaboration (2000) Organised inpatient (stroke unit) care for stroke (Cochrane Review). In: The Cochrane Library, Issue 2. Oxford, Update Software.
2. Powell J, Heslin J, Greenwood R (2002) Community based rehabilitation after severe traumatic brain injury: a randomised controlled trial. J Neurol Neurosurg Psychiatry 72: 193–202.
3. Badley EM (1993) An introduction to the concepts and classifications of the international classification of impairments, disabilities, and handicaps. Disabil Rehabil 15: 161–78.
4. International Classification of Functioning, Disability and Health. World Health Organization.
   http://www3.who.int/icf/icftemplate.cfm.
5. National Health Service Executive (1997) Rehabilitation – A Guide. NHSE, London.
6. Nocon A, Baldwin S (1998) Trends in Rehabilitation Policy – A Literature Review. London, King's Fund.
7. Wade DT (1992) Measurement in Neurological Rehabilitation. Oxford, Oxford University Press.

8. Turner-Stokes L, Williams H, Abraham R, Duckett S (2000) Clinical standards for inpatient specialist rehabilitation services in the UK. Clin Rehabil 14: 468–80.

9. Forbes A, While A, Dyson L et al. (2003) Impact of clinical nurse specialists in multiple sclerosis – synthesis of the evidence. J Adv Nurs 42: 442–62.

10. Hill MC, Johnson J (1999) An exploratory study of nurses' perceptions of their role in neurological rehabilitation. Rehabil Nurs 24: 152–7.

11. MS Trust (2006) Therapists in MS: delivering the long term solutions. London, MS Trust.

12. College of Occupational Therapists (2004) Definition and core skills for occupational therapy. London, College of Occupational Therapists.

13. Yorkston K, Miller R, Strand E et al. (2003) Management of Speech and Swallowing Disorders in Degenerative Disease, 2nd edn. Austin, TX: Pro-Ed.

14. Physiotherapy Explained. Chartered Society of Physiotherapy website. [Cited 16 November 2005]. Available from: www.csp.org.uk.

15. Shepherd G (1990) Case management. Health Trends 22: 59–61.

16. Wade DT, de Jong BA (2000) Recent advances in rehabilitation. BMJ 320: 1385–8.

17. Cunningham C, Horgan F, Keane N et al. (1996) Detection of disability by different members of an interdisciplinary team. Clin Rehabil 10: 247–54.

18. Locke EA, Latham GP (2002) Building a practically useful theory of goal setting and task motivation. A 35-year odyssey. Am Psychol 57: 705–17.

19. Latham GP, Locke EA (1975) Increasing the productivity with decreasing the time limits: a field replication of Parkinson's law. J Appl Psychol 60: 524–6.

20. Yukl GA, Latham GP (1978) Interrelationships among employee participation, individual differences, goal difficulty, goal acceptance, goal instrumentality and performance. Personnel Psychol 31: 305–23.

21. Brown TC, Latham GP (2000) The effects of goal setting and self-instruction training on the performance of unionized employees. Industrial Relations 55: 80–94.

22. Everaert P, Bruggeman W (2002) Cost targets and time pressure during new product development. Int J Operations Product Manage 22: 1339–53.

23. Elliot AJ, Harackiewicz JM (1994) Goal setting: achievement orientation, and intrinsic motivation: a mediational analysis. J Pers Soc Psychol 66: 968–80.

24. Williams KJ, Donovan JJ, Dodge TL (2000) Self regulation of perfor-
    mance; goal establishment and goal revision processes in athletes.
    Hum Perform 13: 159–80.
25. Mone MA, Baker DD (1992) A social–cognitive, attributional model
    of personal goals: an empirical evaluation. Motivation Emotion 16:
    297–321.
26. Schank RC, Fano A, Bell B, Jona M (1994) The design of goal-based
    scenarios. J Learn Sci 3: 305–45.
27. Locke EA (1968) Toward a theory of task motivation and incentives.
    Organ Behav Hum Perform 3: 157–89.
28. Locke EA, Latham GP (1990) The Theory of Goal Setting and Task
    Performance. Englewood Cliffs, NJ, Prentice Hill.
29. Locke EA, Chah D, Harrison S, Lustgarten N (1989) Separating the
    effects of goal specificity from goal level. Organ Behav Hum Perform
    43: 270–87.
30. Dachler HP, Wilpert B (1978) Conceptual dimensions and bound-
    aries of participation in organizations: a critical evaluation. Am Sci
    Q 23: 1–39.
31. Tjosvold D (1988) Co-operative and competitive dynamics within
    and between organisational units. Hum Relations 41: 425–36.
32. Tjosvold D, Andrew I, Struthers J (1992) Leadership influence: goal
    interdependence and power. J Soc Psychol 132: 39–50.
33. Early P, Wojnaroski P, Prest W (1987) Task planning and energy
    expanded: exploration of how goals influence performance. J Appl
    Psychol 72: 107–14.
34. Schut HA, Stam HJ (1994) Goals in rehabilitation teamwork. Disabil
    Rehabil 16: 223–6.
35. Stenstrom CH (1994) Home exercise in rheumatoid arthritis
    functional class II: goal setting versus pain attention. J Rheumatol 21:
    627–34.
36. Webb PM, Glueckauf RL (1994) The effects of direct involvement in
    goal setting on rehabilitation outcome for persons with traumatic
    brain injuries. Rehab Psychol 39: 179–88.
37. Gauggel S, Billino J (2002) The effects of goal setting on the arith-
    metic performance of brain-damaged patients. Arch Clin
    Neuropsychol 17: 283–94.
38. Trombly CA, Radomski MV, Trexel C, Burnet-Smith SE (2002)
    Occupational therapy and achievement of self-identified goals by
    adults with acquired brain injury: phase II. Am J Occup Ther 56:
    489–98.
39. Rossiter D, Thompson AJ (1995) Introduction of integrated care
    pathways for patients with multiple sclerosis in an inpatient neuro-
    rehabilitation setting. Disabil Rehabil 17: 443–8.
40. Edwards SG, Thompson AJ, Playford ED (2004) Integrated care
    pathways: disease-specific or process-specific? Clin Med 4: 132–5.

41. Rossiter DA, Edmondson A, al-Shahi R, Thompson AJ (1998) Integrated care pathways in multiple sclerosis rehabilitation: completing the audit cycle. Mult Scler 4: 85–9.

42. Leary SM, Thompson AJ (2000) Current management of multiple sclerosis. Int J Clin Pract 54: 161–9.

43. MS Society (2002) Developing MS Healthcare Standards: evidence-based recommendations for service providers. London, MS Society.

44. Stuifbergen AK, Becker H, Blozis S et al. (2003) A randomized clinical trial of a wellness intervention for women with multiple sclerosis. Arch Phys Med Rehabil 84: 467–76.

45. Schwarz S, Leweling H (2005) Multiple sclerosis and nutrition. Mult Scler 11: 24–32.

46. Rietberg MB, Brooks D, Uitdehaag BM, Kwakkel G (2005) Exercise therapy for multiple sclerosis. Cochrane Database Syst Rev 1: CD003980.

47. Carter P, White CM (2003) The effect of a general exercise training on effort of walking in patients with multiple sclerosis. 14th International World Confederation for Physical Therapy, Barcelona.

48. DeBolt LS, McCubbin JA (2004) The effects of home-based resistance exercise on balance, power, and mobility in adults with multiple sclerosis. Arch Phys Med Rehabil 85: 290–7.

49. Jones R, Davies-Smith A, Harvey L (1999) The effect of weighted leg raises and quadriceps strength, EMG and functional activities in people with multiple sclerosis. Physiotherapy 3: 154–61.

50. O'Connell R, Murphy RM, Hutchinson M et al. (2003) A controlled study to assess the effects of aerobic training on patients with multiple sclerosis. 14th International World Confederation for Physical Therapy, Barcelona.

51. Petajan JH, Gappmaier E, White AT et al. (1996) Impact of aerobic training on fitness and quality of life in multiple sclerosis. Ann Neurol 39: 432–41.

52. Wiles CM, Newcombe RG, Fuller KJ et al. (2001) Controlled randomised crossover trial of the effects of physiotherapy on mobility in chronic multiple sclerosis. J Neurol Neurosurg Psychiatry 70: 174–9.

53. National Collaborating Centre of Chronic Conditions (2003) Multiple Sclerosis: Management of Multiple Sclerosis in Primary and Secondary Care. Clinical Guideline 8. London, National Institute of Clinical Excellence.

54. Chataway J, Porter B, Heaney D et al. (2005) 'Home or away? A randomised controlled trial of treating acute multiple sclerosis relapses with intravenous steroids. National Hospital for Neurology and Neurosurgery, and Jeremy Hobart, Peninsula Medical School. London, Multiple Sclerosis Society of United Kingdom and Northern Ireland.

55. Lublin FD, Baier M, Cutter G (2003) Effect of relapses on development of residual deficit in multiple sclerosis. Neurology 61: 1528–32.

56. Bethoux F, Miller DM, Kinkel RP (2001) Recovery following acute exacerbations of multiple sclerosis: from impairment to quality of life. Mult Scler 7: 137–42.

57. Craig J, Young CA, Ennis M et al. (2003) A randomised controlled trial comparing rehabilitation against standard therapy in multiple sclerosis patients receiving intravenous steroid treatment. J Neurol Neurosurg Psychiatry 74: 1225–30.

58. Liu C, Playford ED, Thompson AJ (2003) Does neurorehabilitation have a role in relapsing–remitting multiple sclerosis J Neurol 250: 1214–8.

59. Freeman JA, Langdon DW, Hobart JC, Thompson AJ (1997) The impact of inpatient rehabilitation on progressive multiple sclerosis. Ann Neurol 42: 236–44.

60. Freeman JA, Langdon DW, Hobart JC, Thompson AJ (1999) Inpatient rehabilitation in multiple sclerosis: do the benefits carry over into the community? Neurology 52: 50–6.

61. Solari A, Filippini G, Gasco P et al. (1999) Physical rehabilitation has a positive effect on disability in multiple sclerosis patients. Neurology 52: 57–62.

62. Patti F, Ciancio MR, Reggio E et al. (2002) The impact of outpatient rehabilitation on quality of life in multiple sclerosis. J Neurol 249: 1027–33.

63. Patti F, Ciancio MR, Cacopardo M et al. (2003) Effects of a short outpatient rehabilitation treatment on disability of multiple sclerosis patients – a randomised controlled trial. J Neurol 250: 861–6.

64. Lord SE, Wade DT, Halligan PW (1998) A comparison of two physiotherapy treatment approaches to improve walking in multiple sclerosis: a pilot randomized controlled study. Clin Rehabil 12: 477–86.

65. Steultjens EM, Dekker J, Bouter LM et al. (2003) Occupational therapy for multiple sclerosis. Cochrane Database Syst Rev 3: CD003608.

66. MRC (2000) A Framework for Development and Evaluation of RCTs for Complex Interventions to Improve Health. London, MRC.

67. Department of Health (2005) The National Service Framework for long term conditions. London, Department of Health.

68. Wollin JA, Yates PM, Kristjanson LJ (2006) Supportive and palliative care needs identified by multiple sclerosis patients and their families. Int J Palliat Nurs 12: 20–6.

69. NICE (2004) Supportive and palliative care: the Manual. London, NICE.

70. Vaidyanathan S, Soni BM, Gopalan L et al. (1998) A review of the

readmissions of patients with tetraplegia to the Regional Spinal Injuries Centre, Southport, United Kingdom, between January 1994 and December 1995. Spinal Cord 36: 838–46.

71. Royal College of Physicians (1998) Disabled people using hospitals: a charter and guidelines. London, Royal College of Physicians.

4

Managing symptoms in multiple sclerosis

Valerie L Stevenson

Introduction

Over the past decade several immunosuppressant treatments for multiple sclerosis (MS) have become widely available and more including monoclonal antibodies and adhesion molecule therapies are undergoing trials, some of which show promising results. Realistically, however, treatments aimed at reducing disease activity or slowing disease progression will have little or no impact on existing impairments; consequently much of the management of the person with MS will be focused on optimizing function and in the control of symptoms. Appropriate symptom management is essential in aiding rehabilitation and to promote wellbeing. It must, however, be remembered that like other areas of rehabilitation it is important to work with the individual to establish goals of treatment which are functionally relevant and important to them, rather than treating simply at an impairment level. This approach necessitates effective multidisciplinary team working with the individual at all stages to facilitate learning and self-management techniques. As each person with MS has a different experience of any one symptom, there is no uniform management plan applicable to all; instead an individualized approach is required to relieve suffering, to increase comfort and to aid in the optimization of function.

The individual with MS may have input from several different health and social care providers, all of which are responsible for offering their support to enable the individual to incorporate management and treatment strategies into their daily life. As input is from several sources and not from one team or service in isolation, effective communication, co-ordination of management and provision of education and services across health and social care is essential. The majority of the work associated with managing any long-term condition is done in the individual's home and community, with a small fraction of it occurring in the hospital environment.[1,2] It is therefore essential that the person with MS feels they have the knowledge to manage their symptoms effectively and know when and how to seek more specialist input from their health team.

The key to successful symptom management is therefore to ensure the person with MS and, if applicable their family or carers, are educated in self-management techniques and that any interventions are done in an effective and timely fashion. This is a process that is dependent on excellent verbal and written communication with agreed goals and integration of seamless teamwork across health and social care sectors, involving the individual at all stages. Such continuity of care and documentation of the evolving impact of a symptom enables ongoing assessment of change and the appropriate choice and timing of any management intervention. Linking care pathways across healthcare sectors has been identified in recent government publications as one way to promote continuity of quality care.[3–6]

Symptoms in MS may be extremely varied and can co-exist. They may have a detrimental effect on the ability of an individual to continue in employment or education, or impact on fulfilment of life roles including those as a parent or partner. When considering treatment strategies it is often the more 'physical' symptoms that are concentrated on, such as weakness, spasticity, ataxia or sphincter disturbance. However, just as important to the individual are problems such as fatigue, pain, cognitive or sexual dysfunction – symptoms that historically have received less attention and which may be overlooked by the healthcare team. It is therefore important before commencing treatment for any one symptom that all other potential problems are considered. Management plans often include a combination of education, therapy (usually occupational and physiotherapy) and drug treatment, but occasionally there is a place for inpatient rehabilitation or more invasive treatments such as intrathecal baclofen administration for severe spasticity or deep brain stimulation for cerebellar tremor.[7,8]

Spasticity

The impact of spasticity for people with MS is extremely variable, ranging from minor discomfort to devastating loss of function and the development of long-term problems such as pressure sores and contractures. Each individual's experiences are different. Although MS is often considered a disorder of motor function, some people with spasticity or spasms will predominantly describe pain; others experience discomfort or stiffness. Chronic pain or spasms frequently interfere with sleep and can also have an emotional impact on mood, self-image or motivation.[9]

The presence of spasticity or spasms can obviously also impact on function. With regard to mobility, walking may be slower or more difficult, falls more frequent, or the ability to self-propel a wheelchair or transfer compromised. Likewise activities of daily living including washing, dressing, toileting and sexual activity can all be affected. \

Early effective management of spasticity is essential; if poorly managed, serious long-term consequences can occur including muscle shortening and tendon or soft tissue contracture that may lead to restriction of passive movement or physical deformity. Once contractures are present these are often very difficult to modify with long-lasting major functional implications including difficulties carrying out personal hygiene or dressing. With severe contractures, positioning can be affected, predisposing the individual to the development of pressure sores and sometimes resulting in the inability to be seated, which will inevitably lead to restricted community mobility and social isolation.

Despite the contribution of spasticity and spasms to the development of such complications, it is important to remember that the presence of spasticity may actually be useful to the individual, perhaps allowing them to stand or walk when their weakness would not otherwise permit it.

With these issues in mind it is imperative that management is always individualized and function focused rather than simply aimed at the reduction of spasticity as a sign or symptom. The mainstay of management is education of the individual and if applicable their family or carers in strategies to manage their own

Table 4.1. Common cutaneous and visceral stimuli aggravating spasticity[10]

Cutaneous stimuli	Visceral stimuli
Altered skin integrity	Any systemic or localized infection
red or inflamed skin	Bowel dysfunction, e.g. constipation,
broken skin	overflow or diarrhea
infected skin	Bladder dysfunction, e.g. infections,
pressure sores	retention or incomplete emptying
ingrown toenails	Deep vein thrombosis
Tight fitting clothes or urinary	
leg bag straps	
Uncomfortable orthotics or	
seating systems	

spasticity and in the implementation of an effective physical regime including stretching and if possible standing (with or without assistance). One of the key aspects to this education process is ensuring knowledge of the trigger and aggravating factors, detailed in Table 4.1. All of these may exacerbate spasticity and its associated features (spasms, clonus, muscle shortening). Far too often pharmacological treatment for spasticity is escalated before appropriate strategies to manage these factors are instigated.[10] These include bladder and bowel function, skin integrity, soft tissue length and positioning.

Pharmacological measures to treat spasticity

There is no agreed evidence-based model available for the systematic pharmacological management of spasticity, and much of what is done is based on a logical and pragmatic approach. The identification of appropriate treatment goals will help optimize drug therapy in terms of choice of agent but also in timing and dose. For example, painful nocturnal spasms may best be managed with a long-acting agent taken at night-time which has sedative side-effects. Alternatively, stiffness and spasms, which interfere with a person's morning transfers and personal care, may benefit from medication taken on waking prior to the person transferring out of bed. Dosages for individuals who are walking, and who may be relying on their spasticity to do so, are often lower than in those who use a wheelchair for mobility.

A general rule with all medication is to 'start low and go slow'. It may therefore take some time to optimize a treatment regime but this approach will limit any deleterious effects on function or unwanted side-effects. Unfortunately all currently available drug treatments for spasticity can have side-effects, the most commonly reported of which is increased weakness, although it is of course important to recognize that this may actually be as a result of unmasking the degree of underlying weakness by removing tone, which was functionally useful.

Despite optimal nursing, physiotherapy input and the use of physical adjuncts such as specialist seating systems, it is not always possible to control spasticity with a single drug agent without causing unacceptable side-effects. It is therefore preferable to treat an individual with a combination of agents at lower doses to enable effective treatment within the realm of tolerable side-effects.

The oral agents most commonly used to treat spasticity are baclofen, tizanidine, benzodiazepines, dantrolene and gabapentin; all can be used alone as monotherapy or in combination with each other. It is of course also possible to combine oral therapy with local or regional treatments such as botulinum toxin, focal chemical neurolysis or intrathecal therapies including baclofen and phenol.[11]

Baclofen

Baclofen has been evaluated in several studies in MS.[12–14] Most showed a significant change in the Ashworth score with reduced spasms and increased range of motion reported, although none of the studies reported any effect on function. In comparison studies with diazepam, no significant difference in effect was noted but generally patients preferred baclofen due to a reduced side-effect profile.[14]

Side-effects during baclofen treatment may be troublesome and are reported to affect up to 45% of users; they may be a particular problem in the elderly or those with spasticity of cerebral origin who have additional cognitive impairment.[15] Reducing the dose slightly or slowing the rate of dose titration can, however, often moderate them. The most frequently reported effects in clinical trials within the MS population have been sedation, drowsiness, weakness, paresthesia, nausea, vomiting and dry mouth.[14] It is important to note that baclofen should be used with caution in individuals with a history of convulsions as seizure threshold may be reduced with possible loss of control of their epilepsy. Sudden withdrawal should, however, be avoided in all individuals as it may precipitate seizures, confusion, anxiety and hallucinations.[16]

Baclofen is rapidly absorbed through the gastrointestinal tract so its effects can be appreciated quickly; peak plasma levels can occur as soon as 1 hour. It is therefore a useful strategy to administer baclofen half an hour before the clinical effects are particularly wanted, for example getting out of bed in the morning. The half-life is in the order of 3–4 hours so often a three times daily regime is necessary to maintain clinical effectiveness throughout the whole day. The recommended dose range is up to 120 mg daily; higher doses have been reported, although tolerance due to side-effects may be an issue at these levels.[17]

The usual starting dose of baclofen is 5–10 mg daily; it can then be gradually titrated upwards according to effect and tolerance. If side-effects occur it may be necessary to reduce the dosage or slow down the titration. If no benefit is seen at 120 mg daily or maximum tolerated dose then the baclofen should be reduced gradually and withdrawn.

Tizanidine

In comparison to placebo, tizanidine has been shown to reduce muscle tone, frequency of spasms and clonus in people with MS. Like the studies with baclofen no functional benefit has been demonstrated. In comparison studies with diazepam, baclofen and tetrazepam, all drugs appear to be of equal efficacy. Tizanidine had fewer side-effects than diazepam but was comparable to baclofen.[12–14]

Tizanidine is generally well tolerated. The most commonly reported side-effects are sedation, drowsiness, weakness, dry mouth and postural hypotension.

Changes in liver function tests have been documented in subjects taking tizanidine and rare cases of acute fulminant hepatitis have been reported. It is therefore recommended that individuals have their liver function tested before commencement of therapy and then at 2 weeks, 1 month, 3 months and 6 months after, whilst therapy is stabilized.

Tizanidine, like baclofen, is rapidly absorbed through the gastrointestinal tract with peak plasma levels occurring at 1–2 hours. The half-life is in the order of 2–4 hours so a three or even four times daily regimen may be appropriate for individuals. Tizanidine is usually started at a dose of 2 mg daily with increments every few days to a maximum of 36 mg per day.

Dantrolene

Several studies of dantrolene in MS have suggested an improvement in spasticity and spasms; however, none of the trials used validated outcome measures and several were un-blinded.[13,14] In a crossover study comparing dantrolene to diazepam both drugs reduced spasticity and spasms. However, both were associated with significant side-effects; 22 of the 42 patients who completed the study preferred dantrolene, 13 preferred diazepam and seven neither drug.[18]

Unfortunately side-effects are fairly frequent with dantrolene, although they may ameliorate with time. Most commonly reported are gastrointestinal symptoms of anorexia, nausea, vomiting and diarrhea. Additionally there may be some central nervous system effects of drowsiness, fatigue, weakness, dizziness and paresthesia. However, the major limiting factor to its use is the risk of hepatotoxicity.

Acute hepatitis, which may be fatal, is recognized as an idiosyncratic reaction and therefore, like tizanidine, liver function tests are mandatory before initiating therapy and regularly whilst on treatment. The risk of fatal hepatonecrosis is increased in women, those on larger doses (>300 mg a day) or on long-term treatment (>60 days) and those taking concomitant drugs also metabolized in the liver such as estrogens.[19]

The half-life of dantrolene is in the order of 15 hours. Treatment regimes are usually started at a dose of 25 mg once daily and increased gradually by 25 mg increments every few days to a maximum of 100 mg four times a day. The divided dosage regime helps to limit gastrointestinal side-effects.

Benzodiazepines

Most of the studies of diazepam in the management of spasticity have been carried out in people with spinal injuries. In MS most have been comparative studies with other agents (baclofen, tizanidine, ketazolam); these studies have shown similar efficacy between diazepam and the other drugs but an excess of side-effects in the diazepam-treated groups.[14]

Side-effects are frequent and can be divided into central nervous system depressant effects, toxicity and withdrawal syndromes. Most commonly seen are the depressant effects of drowsiness, sedation, reduced attention and memory impairment.

Physiologic dependence can also occur with an associated withdrawal syndrome; therefore benzodiazepines should always be reduced slowly and abrupt cessation of therapy avoided.

Due to the commonest side-effect of sedation, benzodiazepines are often preferred for night-time use only. Clonazepam appears to be particularly useful for nocturnal spasms and stiffness; it can be started at a dose of 0.25–0.5 mg at night. Dose escalation of clonazepam above 1 mg three times a day is rarely tolerated.

Gabapentin

This drug is more commonly prescribed in MS for its beneficial effect on neuropathic pain; however, following some small recent studies it has also gained favor as an anti-spasticity agent where it appears to be a useful adjunct. It may be particularly of value in those individuals who have a combination of pain, spasticity or spasms.

Two small double-blind, placebo-controlled randomized studies have been performed in people with MS[20,21] and another included patients with any cause of upper motor neuron syndrome.[22] All showed a beneficial effect for gabapentin on measures of spasticity.

Generally gabapentin is well tolerated. Its main adverse effects are drowsiness, somnolence and dizziness. The dosage regime does allow for a fairly rapid dose titration. The normal starting dose is 300 mg once a day increasing to 300 mg three times a day by day 3 and then up to a maximum total daily dose of 2400 mg.

There are no significant drug–drug interactions and no necessity to perform blood monitoring.

Cannabinoids

Cannabis has been used by individuals with MS for many years on the basis of anecdotal evidence and on the results of several mostly small studies, which have reported subjective improvement in symptoms of pain, spasms, sleeping, bladder control and spasticity.[23–25]

In a large trial of 630 subjects randomized to either oral placebo, THC (the main active ingredient of the cannabis plant; delta-9-tetrahydrocannabinol) or cannabis extract there was no effect in the primary outcome measure of a change in Ashworth score over the 13-week treatment period.[24] Improvement was seen on patient-reported category rating scales for pain, sleep quality, spasms and spasticity. However, this was in the context of a degree of patient unmasking in the active treatment groups. The conclusion from this study was that, although no major effect on spasticity was noted, some evidence was provided on symptom relief that deserves further attention.[24] Following on from this study, participants were invited to continue study medication (or placebo) in a blinded fashion for up to 1 year. Intention to treat analysis at 12 months revealed a significant beneficial effect on the Ashworth scores of the THC, but not the cannabis extract-treated group.[26]

A further study involved 160 patients who were randomized to either a placebo sublingual spray or a cannabis extract spray. Trial participants recorded a 'primary symptom score' before and after treatment; this was a visual analog score of their worst symptom from a choice of five (spasticity, spasms, pain, bladder dysfunction or tremor). There was no significant difference in these scores between treatment and placebo; however, in the spasticity subset there was a significant treatment effect. No difference was seen in Ashworth scores. As in the first study there was a considerable placebo effect.[23]

The evidence from these studies supports a symptomatic benefit for cannabinoids as well as showing an objective improvement in spasticity as measured by the Ashworth scale for THC-treated individuals in the extended phase of the CAMS study.[24,26] Although not conclusive, this gives further support for a long-term study in MS to assess both symptomatic benefit and impact on disease progression.

The route of administration for pharmaceutical cannabis plant extract or cannabinoids is an important issue. Oral administration is the least efficient mode due to variable plasma levels and significant first-pass metabolism. For this reason sublingual sprays, metered dose inhalers and transdermal patch delivery systems are being proposed as alternative delivery options. The acute side-effects of cannabis are well known. It causes a psychoactive, mildly euphoric state with some psychomotor slowing and cognitive changes particularly impacting on short-term memory.

Anxiety, panic, paranoia and occasional psychosis can also occur. Other effects include appetite stimulation, hypotension, redness of the eyes, dry mouth and dizziness.

Concerns remain over long-term use and the possibility of cognitive impairment and an increased risk of psychosis.[11]

Focal pharmacological therapies

Botulinum toxin is the most widely used treatment for focal spasticity in MS. To maximize the effect of treatment it is essential that botulinum toxin injections be done in conjunction with physiotherapy and/or splinting to obtain the maximum benefit. The toxin is injected directly into the targeted muscle and takes 10–14 days to have a visible effect. As it is reversible, treatment may have to be repeated after a few months although often the introduction of an effective stretching regime is able to maintain the beneficial effects.

There are only two studies specifically assessing the efficacy of botulinum toxin type A in MS, both of which looked specifically at hip adductor tone.[27,28] Both studies showed a significant reduction in spasticity and an improvement in passive function (perineal hygiene). It is relevant, however, that most patients included in these studies were significantly disabled and therefore it is difficult to extrapolate the findings to ambulant individuals who may be more vulnerable to the adverse effect of increased muscle weakness.[14]

Chemical neurolysis by phenol or alcohol is irreversible and results in destruction of neural tissue by protein coagulation. Injections may be targeted at peripheral nerves or motor points (intramuscular injections aimed at the parts of muscle most sensitive to electrical stimulation). Following phenol treatment, partial nerve regeneration and sprouting then occurs so that the clinical effect may 'wear off' after several weeks or months; if necessary the injections can be repeated. Most commonly applied are medial popliteal blocks to aid the spastic drop foot or obturator nerve blocks in either ambulatory patients with scissoring gait or with the aim of improving ease of perineal hygiene and aiding in seating posture.[29]

Intrathecal therapies

If the above measures are not sufficient to manage severe lower limb spasticity then intrathecal baclofen or phenol may be considered. Intrathecal baclofen is delivered by way of a programmable pump implanted into the abdomen, from where a catheter conveys baclofen into the intrathecal space. The dose of baclofen can then be carefully controlled to allow amelioration of spasticity without compromising function. This is particularly important in those individuals who are ambulant.[30]

Occasionally intrathecal baclofen is inappropriate or ineffective in managing severe spasticity causing contracture and inability to seat or hoist an individual safely; these patients may be considered for intrathecal phenol treatment. As phenol is a destructive agent which indiscriminately damages motor and sensory nerves, it is reserved for those individuals who do not have any functional movement in their legs, who have lost bladder and bowel function and who have impaired sensation to their legs. Intrathecal phenol can be an effective treatment which, although it requires expert administration, does not have the long-term maintenance or cost issues that go with intrathecal baclofen treatment. The effect of a single injection often lasts many months and can be repeated if necessary.[9,31]

Ataxia

Cerebellar ataxia is an extremely challenging symptom to manage. The effects on the individual are very variable causing only minor problems with finger dexterity in some but in others catastrophic loss of upper limb function, mobility and even loss of sitting balance. Severe tremor and head titubation may occur and can be very distressing for the individual.

Physiotherapy and occupational therapy is the mainstay of management; through optimizing the individual's seating position, posture and the provision of distal supportive aids, the ease and quality of functional tasks such as feeding, self-care and keyboard use can be considerably improved. Drug therapy is of limited value due to poor efficacy and adverse affects, but occasionally may be helpful. Isoniazid in combination with pyridoxine may have some benefit;[32] other drugs that are often tried with variable success include clonazepam, carbamazepine, mirtazapine and propranolol.[7,33,34] Ondansetron, a 5-HT3 antagonist, has been reported as effective in small studies of patients with severe cerebellar tremor, some of whom had MS. It was well tolerated, the main side-effects being headache and constipation.[35,36]

Cannabinoids and whole plant cannabis extract, despite being advocated by many individuals with MS, has failed to show a benefit for tremor in treatment trials.[23,24,37]

For severe cases of cerebellar tremor or ataxia it may be appropriate to consider neurosurgery. Electrostimulation is most commonly applied to the ventrointeromedial nucleus of the thalamus with a reported 87.7% of patients experiencing at least some sustained improvement in tremor control after surgery.[38] Effects on function have been less consistently reported and preoperative patient education about what functional changes are realistically likely to occur is extremely important.[39] Side-effects may occur and include hemiplegia and dysphagia. Although it is a potentially useful technique, complete cessation of tremor is rarely achieved and frequent reprogramming may be necessary.[38,40]

Pain

Pain in MS is unfortunately common, with incidence rates reported to be between 28.8 and 86% of patients.[14] Most have chronic pain but an estimated 10% have acute paroxysmal pains, the commonest of which is trigeminal neuralgia, which occurs much more often in people with MS than in the general population.[41] It usually responds well to carbamazepine or gabapentin. Other paroxysmal pains also occur including dysesthetic burning pains precipitated by touch, movement or hyperventilation. Painful tonic seizures may be associated with these and may be helped by carbamazepine, gabapentin or lamotrigine.[42–44]

Chronic dysesthetic pain often involves the extremeties.[45] This can be very debilitating for the individual, interfering with mobility and sleep and contributing to depression. The most useful drugs are carbamazepine, gabapentin, pregabalin and the tricyclic antidepressants, particularly amitriptyline. Some of the newer anticonvulsants including lamotrigine, levetiracetam and oxcarbazepine have also shown some benefit in small trials.[45]

Other forms of chronic pain may be secondary to spasticity, or to immobility; back pain is particularly common in wheelchair users. Apart from the effect of immobility and spasticity on the paravertebral musculature, the lumbar area also has to cope with abnormal posturing and often an extremely effortful and abnormal gait; this puts great stress on the spine causing degenerative disease. Early physiotherapy is essential to aid in spasticity management and in the correction of posture and gait, thus limiting further damage. Pain relief should include local measures such as heat pads and transcutaneous electrical nerve stimulation (TENS), although medication such as short-term non-steroidal anti-inflammatory drug use or simple analgesics may be necessary.[7,14]

Bladder and bowel dysfunction

Unfortunately bladder and bowel dysfunction are extremely common in individuals with MS. Estimates of bladder dysfunction are in the order of 75%[46] and bowel dysfunction approximately 50%.[47] Common bladder symptoms are those of frequency, urgency and nocturia. However, as bladder dysfunction increases problems of incontinence, retention and urinary tract infections can all occur. Most of these are a result of a combination of detrusor hyper-reflexia (causing urgency and incontinence) and sphincter dyssynergia (causing failure to empty and frequency, with residual volumes predisposing to infection).[48] Due to the often mixed etiology of urinary symptoms it is essential to assess bladder emptying by measuring the post-micturition residual volume before initiating any therapy; this can be done by either catheterization or transabdominal ultrasound.[49] If there is no residual then detrusor hyper-reflexia can be treated with anticholinergic agents such as oxybutynin or tolterodine. If nocturia fails to be controlled with anticholinergics the use of desmopressin (DDAVP) delivered by a nasal spray can be considered, although caution must be taken to avoid overdose and potentially dangerous hyponatremia.[50] Other potential agents to reduce detrusor hyper-reflexia include intra-vesical capsaicin[51] or botulinum toxin. Two studies of botulinum toxin type A in MS have demonstrated improvements in urodynamics, reduction in incontinence rates and beneficial effects on quality of life with no safety concerns.[52,53]

Detrusor sphincter dyssynergia can be managed using clean, intermittent self-catheterization (CISC). Often by using a combination of CISC and medication bladder control can be markedly improved. Occasionally control remains poor and an indwelling catheter needs to be considered; if this is long term a suprapubic catheter is usually preferred.

Cannabis for bladder dysfunction has been assessed in one small open-label study[54] and as part of larger trials for symptom control in MS.[23,24] Although no significant effects were seen in the larger studies the open-label study demonstrated a significant reduction in frequency, nocturia and incontinence; however, total voided volumes also decreased. There were few side-effects suggesting cannabis-based medicines may be a useful addition to the current treatment armament, though further trials are awaited.[54]

Bowel dysfunction is less frequent than urinary dysfunction but still affects a significant proportion of people with MS and can be extremely distressing. Most commonly individuals complain of constipation and urgency; incontinence is less frequent. Management is more difficult than bladder dysfunction, but the establishment of a routine is important. Often treatment with oral agents used regularly is enough (lactulose, senna, movicol) but glycerine suppositories and micro-enemas can be extremely useful. Incontinence often linked to urgency can be helped with loperamide.[48,55]

Sexual dysfunction

Sexual dysfunction is a problem often overlooked by health professionals but is extremely common; in males with MS the incidence of erectile dysfunction is in the order of 70%.[56] It is usually related to spinal cord involvement and often the occurrence of sexual dysfunction follows on from the development of urinary problems.[48]

Apart from erectile dysfunction, failure to achieve orgasm and ejaculatory difficulties may also occur in men. Psychosexual counseling should be considered in all cases alone or in combination with other therapies. The advent of the phosphodiesterase 5 inhibitors such as sildenafil, tadalafil and vardenafil which are fast-acting oral drugs have reduced the need for more invasive techniques such as intracavernosal injection of alphaprostadil (prostaglandin E_1).[48]

Women complain most frequently of decreased libido, vaginal dryness and of difficulty reaching orgasm. The use of lubricating gels may be helpful and there is some evidence that sildenafil may help some individuals, although the response is less clear than in men.[48,57]

Fatigue

Fatigue may be a particular problem for individuals with MS and is often identified as the single most important symptom interfering with everyday life; if severe it may limit education, employment and social opportunities.[8,58] It may occur at any stage of the disease trajectory and is often increased at times of relapse.

Initial therapy for all causes of fatigue should be aimed at optimizing sleep and the person's general daily routine. For example, treating nocturnal spasms, nocturia, pain or depression may be enough to establish a normal sleeping pattern and reduce daytime fatigue. Occupational therapists and/ or physiotherapists can be of help in devising personalized fatigue management programs which include looking at the individual's daily routine to incorporate energy conservation strategies as well as considering some form of regular exercise, something which has been shown to increase general fitness and reduce fatigue.[59,60]

As fatigue has been recognized as being worse at times of relapse or increased inflammation, it has been hypothesized that, by treating MS with disease-modifying treatments aimed at reducing inflammation, fatigue should improve. This was studied in a cohort of 218 patients treated with either glatiramer acetate or with interferon-β over a 6-month period. Data were collected using the Fatigue Impact Scale. The study was not randomized or double-blind but did suggest that immunomodulatory treatment, specifically glatiramer acetate, may improve MS fatigue.[35]

If necessary, pharmacological measures can be used to directly target MS-related fatigue; the two main agents used are amantadine and modafinil. Both have been shown in small studies to be of some benefit. Central nervous system stimulants such as pemoline are best avoided due to side-effects and dependency. Other agents such as 3,4-diaminopyridine have been investigated but again side-effects are a limiting factor for routine clinical use.[58]

Visual dysfunction

Visual dysfunction in MS can be secondary to lesions in the optic nerves, or in any part of the visual pathway including the occipital cortex or nuclear connections in the brainstem. Common symptoms include loss of acuity, diplopia or oscillopsia; field defects or neglect are rarely seen. Poor recovery from optic neuritis is the commonest cause of visual problems in MS, although brainstem dysfunction causing diplopia, nystagmus and oscillopsia can be very disabling. All patients should be assessed by an optometrist and individuals with optic nerve dysfunction may be helped by referral to low-vision clinics that can assist with registering them as partially sighted. Simple patching can improve comfort and function in people with diplopia. The management of nystagmus and oscillopsia is often challenging; converging prisms may be of use and several drugs have been reported to help in small cohorts of patients; these include baclofen, valproic acid, trihexyphenidyl, clonazepam, isoniazid, gabapentin, memantine and 4-aminopyridine.[61–67] If pharmacological measures fail then retrobulbar botulinum toxin injections can be considered; some benefit has been demonstrated, particularly in patients with severe longstanding oscillopsia.[68]

Speech and swallowing dysfunction

Dysarthria is the most common impairment of communication for people with MS. Often people are able to communicate effectively with friends or relatives who have become accustomed to their speech; however, the input of a speech and language therapist can be invaluable in improving satisfaction and intelligibility. Training in techniques to increase orofacial strength and co-ordination through appropriate exercises, attention to respiratory support to improve phonation and voice quality, and advice on mechanisms to improve intelligibility through altering articulation, speed and prosodic features may all be helpful. If very severe the use of communication aids can also be explored by the therapist. Dysphasia is rare in MS although it may be a feature of atypical large dominant hemisphere lesions.

Swallowing difficulties may be independent of speech problems and can occur in the acute setting of a relapse or insidiously during the progressive phase of the condition where the incidence is probably underestimated.[69] Many individuals will describe fluctuations in their swallow according to factors such as the time of day, temperature and general fatigue. The speech therapist is able to provide education to the individual and if applicable carers in compensatory mechanisms such as posture (tucking the chin in or turning the head) or change in diet. Education should include the dangers of aspiration with advice on how to identify this. If swallowing becomes severely compromised a percutaneous gastrostomy should be considered; although often dreaded by patients and carers, quality of life can be significantly improved.

Mood and cognitive dysfunction

Cognitive dysfunction can be a prominent feature in MS where it is unrelated to disease duration or to level of physical disability. The prevalence has been reported to be in the order of 54–65% in hospital-based studies, and 40% in a large community-based study.[7,70] The pattern of cognitive decline in MS is predominantly subcortical; with the main deficits being in short-term memory, attention, conceptual reasoning and speed of processing.

Cognitive impairment can have a devastating impact on psychosocial functioning. For example, 50–80% of people with MS are unemployed within 10 years of disease onset despite lower than expected levels of physical disability to explain this.[71] By identifying and assessing the nature and extent of cognitive deficits, appropriate strategies to minimize the impact can be developed. Assessment by a neuropsychologist is useful in defining the extent of any dysfunction in domains including memory, attention, speed of processing, language and executive function. Current perfor-mance is compared to an estimate of pre-morbid function. This can be assessed via a test of reading (National Adult Reading Test or NART) or estimated by their previous level of education and employment. Once assessment is complete targeted cognitive rehabilitation programs can be tailored to the individual and if appropriate in conjunction with their employer.[72,73]

People with MS may also develop mood disorders or other psychiatric symptoms. These are usually mild and commonly include low mood, irritability, poor concentration and anxiety.[74] Rates of depression in community samples have ranged between 25 and 41% and tend to be higher in nursing home settings.[75] In addition the majority of people with MS (73%) are reported to have some difficulty controlling emotion with, for example, uncontrolled crying or laughter.[76] Psychological support or cognitive behavioral therapy is often sufficient to manage such symptoms, though if medication is indicated it should be used as in the normal popula-tion but with greater attention to possible adverse effects, particu-larly exacerbation of bladder or sexual dysfunction.

Conclusion

Although great advances have been made in MS management over recent years, there is still a specific need for effective symptom management and rehabilitation for individuals with MS at all stages of their condition. Much can be done to help the individual manage their symptoms from effective and timely education to the input of specialist therapists, pharmacological measures and occasionally more invasive techniques including surgery.

The input of a multidisciplinary team is essential to ensure appropriate input is provided in a co-ordinated and effective manner. As each person with MS has a unique experience and impact of any one symptom, there is no uniform management plan available and an individualized approach is always needed to successfully solve problems and aid in the optimization of function.

The key to successful symptom management is therefore to ensure the person with MS is central to the management process and is actively involved in monitoring the impact of symptoms and in the effectiveness of therapeutic interventions.

References

1. Corbin JM (1998) The Corbin and Strauss Chronic Illness Trajectory model: an update. Sch Inquiry Nurs Pract 12: 33–41.
2. Corbin JM, Strauss A (1991) A nursing model for chronic illness management based upon the trajectory framework. Sch Inquiry Nurs Pract 5: 155–74.
3. Department of Health (2005) Self Care – A Real Choice. London, Central Office of Information (COI). http://www.coi.gov.uk/aboutcoi.php
4. Department of Health (2005) Supporting People with Long Term Conditions. An NHS and social care model to support local innovation and integration. London, Central Office of Information (COI) http://www.coi.gov.uk/aboutcoi.php.
5. Department of Health (2005) National Service frameworks for long-term conditions. London, Department of Health.
6. National Institute of Clinical Excellence Guidelines (2003) Management of Multiple Sclerosis in primary and secondary care. London, NICE.
7. Stevenson VL, Thompson AJ (1998) The management of multiple sclerosis; current and future therapies. Drugs Today 34: 267–82.
8. Kesselring J, Beer S (2005) Symptomatic therapy and neurorehabilitation in multiple sclerosis. Lancet Neurol 74: 643–52.
9. Thompson AJ, Jarrett L, Lockley L et al. (2005) Clinical management of spasticity. J Neurol Neurosurg Psychiatry 76: 459–63.
10. Jarrett L (2006) Provision of education and self-management. In: Stevenson VL, Jarrett L, eds. Spasticity Management: A Practical Multidisciplinary Guide. London, Taylor and Francis.

11. Stevenson VL (2006) Oral medication. In: Stevenson VL, Jarrett L, eds. Spasticity Management: A Practical Multidisciplinary Guide. London, Taylor and Francis.
12. Paisley S, Beard S, Hunn A et al. (2002) Clinical effectiveness of oral treatments for spasticity in multiple sclerosis: a systematic review. Mult Scler 8: 319–29.
13. Shakespeare DT, Boggild M, Young C (2001) Anti-spasticity agents for multiple sclerosis. Cochrane Database Syst Rev 4: CD001332.
14. Beard S, Hunn A, Wight J (2003) Treatments for spasticity and pain in multiple sclerosis: a systematic review. Health Technol Assess 7: 40.
15. Hattab JR (1980) Review of European clinical trials with baclofen. In: Feldman RG, Young RR, Koella WP, eds. Spasticity: Disordered Motor Control. Chicago, Year Book: 71–85.
16. Terrence DV, Fromm GH (1981) Complications of baclofen withdrawal. Arch Neurol 38: 588–9.
17. Smith CR, La Rocca NG, Giesser BS et al. (1991) High-dose oral baclofen: experience in patients with multiple sclerosis. Neurology 41: 1829–31.
18. Schmidt RT, Lee RH, Spehlmann R (1976) Comparison of dantrolene sodium and diazepam in the treatment of spasticity. J Neurol Neurosurg Psychiatry 39: 350–6.
19. Pinder RM, Brogden RN, Speight TM et al. (1977) Dantrolene sodium: a review of its pharmacological properties and therapeutic effect in spasticity. Drugs 13: 3–23.
20. Mueller ME, Gruenthal M, Olson WL et al. (1997) Gabapentin for relief of upper motor neuron symptoms in multiple sclerosis. Arch Phys Med Rehabil 78: 521–4.
21. Cutter NC, Scott DD, Johnson JC et al. (2000) Gabapentin effect on spasticity in multiple sclerosis: a placebo-controlled, randomized trial. Arch Phys Med Rehabil 81: 164–9.
22. Formica A, Verger K, Sol JM et al. (2005) Gabapentin for spasticity: a randomized, double-blind, placebo-controlled trial. Med Clin (Barc) 124: 81–5.
23. Wade DT, Makela P, Robson P et al. (2004) Do cannabis-based medicinal extracts have general or specific effects on symptoms in multiple sclerosis? A double-blind, randomized, placebo-controlled study on 160 patients. Mult Scler 10: 434–41.
24. Zajicek J, Fox P, Sanders H (2003) Cannabinoids for treatment of spasticity and other symptoms related to multiple sclerosis (CAMS study): multicentre randomised placebo-controlled trial. Lancet 362: 1517–26.
25. Vaney C, Heinzel-Gutenbrunner M, Jobin P et al. (2004) Efficacy, safety and tolerability of an orally administered cannabis extract in the treatment of spasticity in patients with multiple sclerosis: a randomized, double-blind, placebo-controlled, crossover study. Mult Scler 10: 417–42.

26. Zajicek JP, Sanders HP, Wright DE et al. (2005) Cannabinoids in multiple sclerosis (CAMS) study: safety and efficacy data for 12 months follow-up. J Neurol Neurosurg Psychiatry 76: 1664–9.

27. Snow BJ, Tsui JKC, Bhatt MH et al. (1990) Treatment of spasticity with botulinum toxin: a double blind study. Ann Neurol 28: 512–15.

28. Hyman N, Barnes M, Bhakta B et al. (2000) Botulinum toxin (Dysport) treatment of hip adductor spasticity in multiple sclerosis: a prospective, randomised, double blind, placebo controlled, dose ranging study. J Neurol Neurosurg Psychiatry 68: 707–12.

29. Barnes MP (1993) Local treatment of Spasticity. Baillières Clin Neurol 2: 55–71.

30. Jarrett L, Leary SM, Porter B et al. (2001) Managing spasticity in people with multiple sclerosis. A goal orientated approach to intrathecal baclofen therapy. Int J MS Care 3: 2–11.

31. Jarrett L, Nandi P, Thompson AJ (2002) Managing severe lower limb spasticity in multiple sclerosis: does intrathecal phenol have a role? J Neurol Neurosurg Psychiatry 73: 705–9.

32. Hallett M, Lindsey JW, Adelstein BD et al. (1985) Controlled trial of isoniazid therapy for severe postural cerebellar tremor in multiple sclerosis. Neurology 35: 1374–7.

33. Alusi SH, Worthington J, Glickman S et al. (2001) A study of tremor in multiple sclerosis. Brain 124: 720–30.

34. Thompson AJ (2002) Progress in neurorehabilitation in multiple sclerosis. Curr Opin Neurol 15: 267–70.

35. Metz L, Hinrichs J, Harris C (1996) Assessment of oral ondansetron in the treatment of cerebellar tremor in MS using the Canadian Occupational Performance Measure. MS Clin Lab Res 2: 116.

36. Rice GP, Ebers GC (1995) Ondansetron for intractable vertigo complicating acute brainstem disorders. Lancet 345: 1182–83.

37. Fox P, Bain PG, Glickman S et al. (2004) The effect of cannabis on tremor in patients with multiple sclerosis. Neurology 62: 1105–9.

38. Wishart HA, Roberts DW, Roth RM et al. (2003) Chronic deep brain stimulation for the treatment of tremor in multiple sclerosis: review and case reports. J Neurol Neurosurg Psychiatry 74: 1392–7.

39. Berk C, Carr J, Sinden M et al. (2002) Thalamic deep brain stimulation for the treatment of tremor due to multiple sclerosis: a prospective study of tremor and quality of life. J Neurosurg 97: 815–20.

40. Geny C, Nguyen JP, Pollin B et al. (1996) Improvement of severe postural cerebellar tremor in multiple sclerosis by chronic thalamic stimulation. Mov Disord 11: 489–94.

41. Manzoni GC, Torelli P (2005) Epidemiology of typical and atypical craniofacial neuralgias. Neurol Sci 26(Suppl 2): S65–7.

42. Espir ML, Millac P (1970) Treatment of paroxysmal disorders in multiple sclerosis with carbamazepine (Tegretol). J Neurol Neurosurg Psychiatry 33: 528–31.

43. Solaro C, Lunardi GL, Capello E et al. (1998) An open-label trial of gabapentin treatment of paroxysmal symptoms in multiple sclerosis patients. Neurology 51: 609–11.
44. Cianchetti C, Zuddas A, Randazzo AP et al. (1999) Lamotrigine adjunctive therapy in painful phenomena in MS: preliminary observations. Neurology 53: 433.
45. Irving GA (2005) Contemporary assessment and management of neuropathic pain. Neurology 64(Suppl 3): S21–S27.
46. Betts CD, D'Mellow MT, Fowler CJ (1993) Urinary symptoms and the neurological features of bladder dysfunction in multiple sclerosis. J Neurol Neurosurg Psychiatry 56: 245–50.
47. Chia YW, Fowler CJ, Kamm MA et al. (1995) Prevalence of bowel dysfunction in patients with multiple sclerosis and bladder dysfunction. J Neurol 242: 105–8.
48. DasGupta R, Fowler CJ (2003) Bladder, bowel and sexual dysfunction in multiple sclerosis: management strategies. Drugs 63: 153–66.
49. Fowler CJ (1996) Investigation of the neurogenic bladder. J Neurol Neurosurg Psychiatry 60: 6–13.
50. Eckford SD, Carter PG, Jackson SR et al. (1995) An open, in-patient incremental safety and efficacy study of desmopressin in women with multiple sclerosis and nocturia. Br J Urol 76: 459–63.
51. Fowler CJ, Beck RO, Gerrard S et al. (1994) Intravesical capsaicin for treatment of detrusor hyperreflexia. J Neurol Neurosurg Psychiatry 57: 169–73.
52. Schurch B, de Seze M, Denys P et al. (2005) Botulinum toxin type a is a safe and effective treatment for neurogenic urinary incontinence: results of a single treatment, randomized, placebo controlled 6–month study. J Urol 174: 196–200.
53. Gallien P, Reymann JM, Amarenco G et al. (2005) Placebo controlled, randomised, double blind study of the effects of botulinum A toxin on detrusor sphincter dyssynergia in multiple sclerosis patients. J Neurol Neurosurg Psychiatry 76: 1670–6.
54. Brady CM, DasGupta R, Dalton C et al. (2004) An open-label pilot study of cannabis-based extracts for bladder dysfunction in advanced multiple sclerosis. Mult Scler 10: 425–33.
55. Wald A (1994) Pathophysiology and management of fecal incontinence. Rev Gastroenterol Mex 59: 139–46.
56. Zorzon M, Zivadinov R, Bosco A et al. (1999) Sexual dysfunction in multiple sclerosis: a case–control study. I. Frequency and comparison of groups. Mult Scler 5: 418–27.
57. DasGupta R, Wiseman OJ, Kanabar G et al. (2004) Efficacy of sildenafil in the treatment of female sexual dysfunction due to multiple sclerosis. J Urol 171: 1189–93.
58. Krupp LB (2003) Fatigue in multiple sclerosis: definition, pathophysiology and treatment. CNS Drugs 17: 225–34.

59. Mathiowetz VG, Finlayson ML, Matuska KM et al. (2005) Randomized controlled trial of an energy conservation course for persons with multiple sclerosis. Mult Scler 11: 592–601.

60. Petajan JH, Gappmaier E, White AT et al. (1996) Impact of aerobic training on fitness and quality of life in multiple sclerosis. Ann Neurol 39: 432–41.

61. Averbuch-Heller L, Stahl JS, Rottach KG et al. (1995) Gabapentin as treatment of nystagmus. Ann Neurol 38: 972.

62. Currie JN, Matsuo V (1986) The use of clonazepam in the treatment of nystagmus-induced oscillopsia. Ophthalmology 93: 924–32.

63. Herishanu Y, Louzoun Z (1986) Trihexyphenidyl treatment of vertical pendular nystagmus. Neurology 36: 82–4.

64. Lefkowitz D, Harpold G (1985) Treatment of ocular myoclonus with valproic acid. Ann Neurol 17: 103–4.

65. Starck M, Albrecht H, Pollmann W et al. (1997) Drug therapy for acquired pendular nystagmus in multiple sclerosis. J Neurol 244: 9–16.

66. Straube A (2005) Pharmacology of vertigo/nystagmus/oscillopsia. Curr Opin Neurol 18: 11–14.

67. Traccis S, Rosati G, Monaco MF et al. (1990) Successful treatment of acquired pendular elliptical nystagmus in multiple sclerosis with isoniazid and base-out prisms. Neurology 40: 492–4.

68. Repka MX, Savino PJ, Reinecke RD (1994) Treatment of acquired nystagmus with botulinum neurotoxin A. Arch Ophthalmol 112: 1320–4.

69. Hughes JC, Enderby PM, Hewer RL (1994) Dysphagia and multiple sclerosis: a study and discussion of its nature and impact. Clin Rehabil 8: 18–26.

70. Rao SM, Leo GJ, Bernardin L et al. (1991) Cognitive dysfunction in multiple sclerosis. I. Frequency, patterns, and prediction. Neurology 41: 685–91.

71. Rao SM, Leo GJ, Ellington L et al. (1991) Cognitive dysfunction in multiple sclerosis. II. Impact on employment and social functioning. Neurology 41: 692–6.

72. Bagert B, Camplair P, Bourdette D (2002) Cognitive dysfunction in multiple sclerosis: natural history, pathophysiology and management. CNS Drugs 16: 445–55.

73. Langdon DW, Thompson AJ (1996) Cognitive problems in multiple sclerosis. MS Management 3: 1,6–9.

74. Ron MA, Logsdail SJ (1989) Psychiatric morbidity in multiple sclerosis: a clinical and MRI study. Psychol Med 19: 887–95.

75. Rickards H (2005) Depression in neurological disorders: Parkinson's disease, multiple sclerosis, and stroke. J Neurol Neurosurg Psychiatry 76: 48–52.

76. Feinstein A, O'Connor P, Gray T et al. (1999) Pathological laughing and crying in multiple sclerosis: a preliminary report suggesting a role for the prefrontal cortex. Mult Scler 5: 69–73.

5

Measuring multiple sclerosis rehabilitation outcomes

Stefan J Cano and Jeremy C Hobart

Introduction

In recent years, the importance of evaluating the impact of multiple sclerosis (MS) rehabilitation has become clear. However, health cannot be measured directly and instead indicators are used to represent clinical outcomes. Increasingly, rating scales are used to score aspects of disease or elicit patients' opinion about aspects of health. To justify their important role in research and clinical practice, measures must be demonstrated to be rigorous indicators of these abstract and unobservable variables.

This chapter provides information on the main issues surrounding the use of rating scales in MS rehabilitation, in particular the science behind the measurement of disease and treatment. It has five aims: (1) to provide a background to psychometrics – the science of measurement; (2) to describe the main tests and criteria for rigorous measurement; (3) to provide information that can be used to evaluate rating scales; (4) to provide the references needed to gain a full appreciation of rating scale science and (5) to provide information on some rating scales in MS rehabilitation.

A history of psychometrics in health measurement

Although health measurement as a distinct discipline emerged in the 1980s,[1-3] it is derived from well-established theories and methods in the social sciences originating from psychophysics in the 1800s. The use of clinical outcome measures can be traced back to the beginning of the 20th century with Ernest Amory Codman, an orthopedic surgeon at the Massachusetts General Hospital, Boston.[4] However, it was not until after the second world war, that rating scales were more widely used in areas such as neurological outcomes,[5] post-procedural complications[6] and physical performance.[7]

Despite the increased use of rating scales in medicine, the use of psychometrics in health measurement did not emerge until the 1970s, when the focus of healthcare evaluation moved from traditional clinical outcomes (i.e. mortality, morbidity) to the measurement of function (i.e. the ability of patients to perform the daily activities of their lives).[8] The shift from traditional outcome measures to the wider encompassing health outcomes measurement occurred for a number of reasons. First, the narrow definition of health in terms of morbidity and mortality was replaced by a broader definition of health as a 'complete state of physical, mental and social well-being and not merely the absence of disease or infirmity'.[9] Second, public health campaigns, rising standards of living, aging populations and the development of health technology led to a shift in attention from the cure of acute diseases to the management of more complex, chronic conditions (e.g. MS, Parkinson's disease). This resulted in an increased interest in measuring more complex and subjective aspects of health outcomes.[10] Third, more demand has come from healthcare trusts for clinicians to demonstrate evidence of cost effectiveness, in which the benefits of a particular health service or intervention are weighed against the costs of that service or intervention.[11] The primary source of this information is standardized surveys,[1] for which psychometric techniques of scale construction are highly appropriate.[8]

Measuring clinical variables

Psychometric methods have been slow to transfer to clinical practice despite its rapid expansion in the health measurement literature since the mid-1980s. This may be due to many clinicians not having time to learn about instrument development and evaluation, and the literature, which is directed primarily towards educationalists and psychologists, may seem incomprehensible.[12] Also, some clinicians have regarded health measurement as 'soft science'[13] which produces 'soft data' (e.g. self-reported functioning, satisfaction with treatment) and often prefer 'hard data' such as tangible variables measured with mechanical instruments (e.g. magnetic resonance imaging (MRI) in MS, mortality rates in stroke, seizure frequency in epilepsy, complications of treatment of cerebral hemorrhage) or clinician judgment, even when these are of limited value in measuring outcome.[14]

There is some evidence that physician-oriented outcomes are not always related to patient-oriented outcomes. Pertinent examples in neurology include the weak relationship between: lesion load quantified by MRI of the brain and disability in MS;[15] seizure frequency and aspects of wellbeing in epilepsy;[16] and tremor severity and physical and mental health in Parkinson's disease.[17] It is not surprising, therefore, that treatments with demonstrated effectiveness in terms of physiological parameters and clinical endpoints are not always associated with a positive impact on health status. For example, although there is incontrovertible evidence that the use of interferon-β in MS reduces abnormalities detected by MRI and relapse rate,[18,19] the effect on disability is unclear and is associated with considerable controversy.[20] In contrast to this, it has been shown that data from self-report rating scales are good predictors of long-term outcome.

One of the most compelling reasons for assessing general perceived health is that it predicts subsequent morbidity and mortality, even after controlling for other biological variables.[21] In a study that measured quality of life (QoL) in patients with advanced breast cancer undergoing chemotherapy, the most accurate predictor of survival was initial QoL scores.[22] These findings have been supported by other studies.[23,24] Thus, 'soft' outcomes are becoming more widely accepted and patients' views and perceptions of their own health are recognized as being an essential part of healthcare evaluation.[25]

What is a rating scale?

There are many methods, termed scaling models, for combining multiple items into rating scales depending on the purpose the resulting scale is to serve.[26-30] The most widely used scaling model in health measurement is the method of summated rating proposed by Likert in 1932.[31,32] Four characteristics constitute a summated rating scale. First, there are multiple items whose scores are summed, without weighting, to generate a total score. Second, each item measures a property that can vary quantitatively (e.g. difficulty walking ranges from none to unable to walk). Third, each item has no right answer. Fourth, each item in the scale can be rated independently. Examples of Likert scales in health measurement are: the Barthel Index (BI);[33] Functional Independence Measure (FIM);[34] Medical Outcomes Study 36-item Short Form Health Survey (SF-36);[35] General Health Questionnaire (GHQ);[36] Hospital Anxiety and Depression Scale (HADS);[37] and the Parkinson's Disease Questionnaire (PDQ-39).[17] Likert scales are popular because they are simple, easy to administer, user friendly, cheap, relatively straightforward to develop, and can be reliable and valid.

Philosophically, rating scales can be classified into two distinct approaches.[38,39] First, the standard needs approach describes measuring health outcomes as the extent to which certain universal needs are met. This approach advocates that there is a standard set of life circumstances that are required for optimal functioning. Although a subjective phenomenon, health outcomes are an objective characteristic of an individual. Second, and in contrast, the psychological processes approach views health outcomes as constructed from individual evaluations of personally salient aspects of life. This approach sees health outcomes as being made up of perception of life circumstances, dependent on the psychological make-up of an individual, rather than on their life circumstances alone. The central assumption of this approach is that each person is the best source of judgments about health outcomes, and one cannot assume that all people will value different circumstances in the same way.

Many types of rating scale can be classed as following the standard needs approach, ranging from generic measures that provide comprehensive, general evaluations of health outcomes, to those that concentrate on a specific aspect of health (e.g. symptoms). The former is illustrated by the SF-36[35] which focuses on activities of daily living (e.g. personal care, domestic roles, mobility) and on role functioning (e.g. work, finance, family, friends and social). Generic measures permit direct comparisons of different patient populations, thereby providing the opportunity to make policy decisions across a variety of diseases.[22] The use of generic measures may enhance the generalizability of a study or help interpret results in a wider context. In addition, it can be argued that generic measures are likely to be robust as they are used and tested in many different settings. However, generic measures may be limited as they may be unable to address important aspects of outcome that are affected by a particular disease, and are generally not sensitive enough to detect changes in outcome which occur in response to treatment or over time.[40]

There are three types of standard needs measures that concentrate on a more specific aspect of health: disease/condition-specific, site-specific and dimension-specific. The most commonly used of these measures are disease/condition-specific measures, which are developed for use in a specific disease or condition. These include items that are directly relevant to the condition and are, therefore, likely to be shorter and appear more appropriate,[22] which helps to reduce patient burden and increase acceptability.[41] Disease-specific measures ensure more comprehensive assessment of important outcome domains, and are generally more sensitive in detecting the effects of treatment on outcome and changes in outcome over time.[22] However, they do not allow comparisons to be made between different patient groups, and it is argued that these instruments may not capture health problems associated with a disease and its treatments that have not been anticipated. In addition, these measures are not always appropriate in studies which include control groups.

Site-specific measures assess health problems in a specific part of the body, such as the Oxford Hip Score.[42] As with disease/condition-specific instruments, these include fewer items and appear more appropriate, which helps to reduce patient burden and increase acceptability. However, it is argued that these instruments may not capture health problems associated with a disease and its treatments that have not been anticipated,[43] and they are unlikely to detect the side-effects of an intervention.

Dimension-specific measures provide comprehensive, general evaluations of one specific aspect of QoL that may be applicable across different patient groups and treatments. Examples of these measures include psychological outcomes (e.g. General Health Questionnaire (GHQ),[36] Hospital Anxiety and Depression

Scale (HADS)).[37] The advantage of such measures is that they provide a more detailed assessment in the area of concern. Many of these instruments are widely used in a range of clinical populations so that there are comparative data. However, the drawback of these measures is that some have been developed for diagnosis or needs assessment and may not be appropriate as outcome measures (e.g. responsive to clinical change).

It is argued that comprehensive assessment of outcome should include a combination of generic and specific measures.[22,40] Generic measures allow comparisons to be made across studies, thus enhancing the generalizability of findings; specific measures provide better content validity, and are generally more responsive due to greater relevance to the specific population.

In contrast to using generic or specific measures with predetermined content, proponents of the psychological processes approach argue that listing items in measurement scales does not capture the subjectivity of human beings and the individual structure of values. In short, prescribing items using a preordained definition of QoL and matching the person to the definition (i.e. 'goodness of fit'), does not let us know whether all the domains, pertinent and meaningful to each respondent, are included. This viewpoint has influenced the development of 'individualized' measures such as the Schedule for the Evaluation of Individual Quality of Life (SEIQoL).[39] This measure allows individuals to nominate important domains of QoL and weight those domains in order of importance. Another measure, the Patient Generated Index (PGI), asks individuals to identify those aspects of life that are personally affected by health.[44] The main advantage of these measures includes a claim for validity as the areas of importance are selected by the individuals involved in completing the measures. The main disadvantages are that some of these measures require trained interviewers, which translates into a need for greater resources, and lower practicality. Also, it is less easy to produce population-based comparative or normative data given the variation in each individual completed measure.[43]

Choosing health rating scales

Neurologists, researchers and clinical trialists often have to choose one scale from among many potential candidates.[45,46] Unfortunately, no one rating scale exhibits all desirable qualities.

Different scales have different virtues, and measures that are useful for one scenario may not be useful for others. Therefore, scales must be selected for the particular purpose for which they are to be used and the scale user must be able to choose measures intelligently based on their needs. Measures must be clinically useful and scientifically sound. Clinical usefulness refers to the successful incorporation of an instrument into clinical practice and its appropriateness to the study sample. Scientific soundness refers to the demonstration of reliable, valid and responsive measurement of the outcome of interest. Clinical usefulness does not guarantee scientific soundness, and vice versa.

When considering the quality of a rating scale we recommend examining at least seven measurement properties: data quality, scaling assumptions, targeting acceptability, reliability, validity and responsiveness.

Measurement properties to consider
Data quality

Indicators of data quality, such as per cent item non-response and per cent computable scores, determine the extent to which an instrument can be incorporated into a clinical setting. These indicators, like all psychometric properties, vary across samples.[47] If the measure is patient-report, these indicators reflect respondents' understanding and acceptance of it and help to identify items that may be irrelevant, confusing, or upsetting to patients.[47] If the measure is clinician-report these indicators reflect the ability to incorporate it into a clinical setting. When there are large amounts of missing data for items, scores for scales cannot be reliably estimated.

Scaling assumptions

Tests of scaling assumptions determine whether it is legitimate to generate scores for an instrument using the algorithms proposed by the developers. For example, the SF-36[35] is a generic measure of health status that has 36 items grouped into eight scales. A score is generated for each SF-36 scale by summing scores across groups of items. However, few investigators examine whether the assumptions that underpin the summing of items to generate scores are satisfied. Items can be summed without weighting or standardization when they measure at the same point on the scale (have similar mean scores), contribute similarly to the variance of the total score (have similar variances), measure a common underlying construct (the items must be internally consistent) and are correctly grouped into scales (hypothesized item groupings are supported by techniques including factor analysis and examination of item convergent and discriminant validity). It is recommended that item-own subscale correlations (corrected for overlap) should exceed item-other subscale correlations by at least two standard errors $(2 \times 1/\sqrt{n})$.[48]

Targeting

Targeting is the extent to which the spectrum of health measured by a scale matches the distribution of health in the study sample and is determined simply by examining score distributions.[49] Ideally, the observed scores from a sample should span the entire range of the scale, the mean score should be near the scale midpoint, and floor and ceiling effects (per cent of the sample having the minimum and maximum score, respectively) should be small. McHorney and Tarlov recommend that floor and ceiling effects should be <15%.[50]

Reliability

The reliability of a measure is the degree to which it is free from random error. Observed scores produced by rating scales are the synthesis of three components: a 'true score' component; a systematic error; and a random error component.[51] It is important to understand the relative contributions of each component. If no random error is present, the reliability is 1.0; this number approaches zero as the relative amount of random error increases. The 'true score' component and systematic error contribute to the reliability of a measure, as they steer the score for an individual towards a consistent value. Systematic error leads to bias, because it causes a score to be consistently too high or too low relative to the true score. Reliability is an important property of a rating scale, because it is essential to establish that any changes observed in patient groups are due to the intervention or disease and not to problems in the measure.[43] In addition, the reliability of a particular measure is not a fixed property, but is dependent upon the situation and patient group studied.[12] In general, there are two approaches commonly used to evaluate the reliability of rating scales. Each reflects different ways of estimating random error: internal consistency and test–retest.

Internal consistency is a function of the number of items and their covariation within a scale measuring a construct (e.g. symptoms, psychological functioning[51]). It can be assessed in a number of different ways. However, Cronbach's coefficient alpha[52] is the most commonly used to estimate the reliability of a measure based on internal consistency. A higher alpha indicates better reliability. However, there are two points of caution regarding misleading interpretations. First, Cronbach's alpha can be increased by increasing the number of items, even if the average level of correlation does not change.[12] The greater the number of items in a scale, the higher the alpha. Second, if items of a scale are very highly intercorrelated, it is likely that there is some redundancy among the items, and also a possibility that the items together are addressing a narrow aspect of the construct. The criterion for adequate reliability is Cronbach's alpha coefficient >0.80.[52]

The second approach commonly used to evaluate reliability is test–retest or reproducibility. This form of reliability assesses whether a measure yields the same results on repeated applications, when respondents have not changed on the construct being measured. Intraindividual response variability is used to estimate random error in test–retest assessments.[51] For continuous data, the Pearson product-moment correlation coefficient or the intraclass correlation coefficient (ICC) are often computed to estimate test–retest reliability, in order to assess the extent to which individuals who scored high on the initial assessment, also tend to score high on the repeated assessment, and vice versa. The intraclass correlation is considered superior to the Pearson correlation coefficient in assessing test–retest reliability, as the former is sensitive to variation in systematic changes in scores as well as the relative ordering of different respondents.[53] The criterion for adequate reliability is ICC ≥0.80.[54]

Validity

In contrast to reliability, validity is, in general, the extent to which an instrument measures what it intends to measure. Validity involves gathering information in the process of developing or using a measure relevant to its specific purpose or set of purposes. Validity can be considered 'an overall evaluative judgment of the degree to which empirical evidence and theoretical rationale support the adequacy and appropriateness of interpretations and actions on the basis of test scores or other modes of assessment' (p741; reference 55). It reflects the appropriateness of inferences made when interpreting a score produced by a measure.[56] Assessing validity is important, as it involves the accumulation of evidence that contributes to defining the meaning of a score.[57] The distinction between reliability and validity is important because a measure may be reliable (i.e. always yield the same score) but may not be valid, as it may be consistently measuring the same thing but not what it is supposed to measure. There are two main types of validity that are particularly relevant to health measurement: content validity and construct validity.

Content validity refers to how well a measure covers important parts of the health components that are required for the measure's intended purpose. There are two main sides to content validity. The first is content relevance, which refers to the specification of the constructs (or domains) in question together with specification of the intended purpose of the measure.[58] The second side to content validity is content coverage, which refers to the specification of procedures for sampling the domain in some representative fashion.[58] In order to evaluate content validity, qualitative methods are used as opposed to statistical criteria, using evidence (e.g. literature, expert opinion, patient views) obtained during the development of the measure.

Construct validity involves specifying the dimensions of a construct, and the expected relations of the dimensions to each other, both internally and externally.[56] Ideally, the relation to external domains would involve using other measures generally accepted as a more accurate or criterion variable. However, in health measurement, it is rare to find perfect gold standard measures against which to evaluate the validity of a new measure. Therefore, construct validity is often used in the absence of criterion variables.

Construct validity is evaluated by hypothesizing how a measure should perform and confirming this hypothesis or not.[51] One of the most common ways to assess this in health measurement is 'convergent and discriminant validity'; the former offers convergent evidence that the measure is related to other measures (or other variables) of the same construct on theoretical grounds, and the latter provides discriminant evidence that the measure is not related to other distinct constructs.[59] Discriminant validity is important in order to discount plausible counter-hypotheses to the interpretation of the construct.[60] Overall, no single observation can prove the construct validity of a new measure; rather it is necessary to build up a picture from a broad pattern of relationships of a new measure with other variables.[55] In fact, construct validity has been described as a never-ending process.[57]

Responsiveness

If a new measure is to be used in evaluating the effects of a given intervention (e.g. interferon-β in MS), the responsiveness of the measure needs to be evaluated. Responsiveness, a type of validity, can be considered as the ability of a measure to detect significant change over time, such as an indication of a therapeutic effect or a meaningful reduction in symptoms from the patient's perspective. It is an essential property of a measure that is used to evaluate change over time. To be useful, the user of a rating scale must know the degree to which a measure can detect differences in outcomes that are important.[53]

There are two major components to responsiveness: 'internal' and 'external'.[61] Internal responsiveness is the ability of the scales of a measure to detect change over a set time period. The three most common ways of calculating this are: effect size,[62] t-test comparisons, and the responsiveness statistic.[63] However, this type of responsiveness only provides a statistically significant change over time, which may not be synonymous with clinically important change.[62] Therefore, 'external responsiveness' is used to reflect the extent to which change in a measure relates to corresponding change in a reference clinical or health status measure. 'External responsiveness' of an instrument can be calculated by comparing to a reference measure that is regarded as an accepted indication of change,[61] and can be expressed in terms of receiver operating characteristics, correlation and regression models. Cohen defined an effect size of 0.20 as small, one of 0.50 as moderate and one of 0.80 or greater as large.[62]

Evaluating scales

If a scale is chosen that has no published evidence concerning its measurement properties, it should be evaluated. The aim of scale evaluation is to determine whether an instrument satisfies criteria for rigorous measurement. Much of this information can be gained from the retrospective analysis of data if they have already been collected. However, prospective studies evaluating the seven measurement properties described above are often required.

Evaluation is important for two reasons. First, the properties of a scale described in the previous section are sample dependent (not simply disease dependent) and, therefore, the performance of a measure in a specific application is more important than its performance generally.[47] Second, data are only as strong as the instruments used to collect them. Sophisticated statistical methods and advances in study design will do little to overcome the damage done by poor-quality measures.[64,65] It is sobering to think that vast amounts of money have been spent evaluating the impact of interferons on disability in MS using a measure, the Expanded Disability Status Scale (EDSS).[66] Prior to these studies there had been limited evaluation of the EDSS using formal psychometric methods. Subsequently evaluations have demonstrated a limited ability to discriminate between individuals and groups known to differ in their levels of disability, and poor responsiveness.[67,68]

Rating scales for MS rehabilitation
Towards rigorous measurement

In MS rehabilitation, it is particularly pertinent to use rating scales to measure outcome, as MS is associated with disablement, is chronic, progressive and associated with little prospect of cure. Moreover, advances in basic neuroscience have resulted in the development of therapeutic interventions that modify disease progression (e.g. interferon-β for MS[69]). Inpatient MS rehabilitation is a therapeutic intervention that provides a co-ordinated multidisciplinary approach to managing the everyday problems of people with disablement associated with neurological diseases. It is recognized as an integral part of healthcare in neurology and advocated as an important and effective intervention.[70]

The inclusion of new rating scales developed using a rigorous psychometric approach has been slow to translate to MS rehabilitation for three main reasons. First, there have been dramatic advances in basic neuroscience, particularly in neuroimaging (MRI), that have maintained the focus on physician-oriented outcomes. Research interest has focused on MRI as an objective measure of treatment effectiveness[71] rather than on patient-oriented measures. Second, the attention has typically focused on the rigor of study design rather than measurement. For example, the MS literature has been more concerned with issues of blinding,[72] randomization,[73] placebo controls,[74] sample size,[75] ethics[76] and data analysis,[77,78] rather than on the development and evaluation of outcome measures. This bias indicates a failure to appreciate that study design is directly dependent on the properties of the instruments used,[64] and that the quality of data is dependent on the quality of the measures used to collect the data.[65] The third and perhaps most important reason for the slow progression of patient-oriented outcome measurement in MS rehabilitation is due to a general lack of awareness of the science of measurement. Although there is an enormous social sciences literature on methods for rigorously measuring complex constructs, it is not surprising that neurologists are generally unfamiliar with the fundamental principals of the science of measurement, as this literature is outside their domain of expertise.

What to measure

As there is no consensus as to how inpatient rehabilitation should be delivered, there are considerable variations in clinical practice.[79–81] However, there is a common conceptual and practical framework to rehabilitation practice that is based on a model of comprehensive care.[82] This model emphasizes that rehabilitation extends beyond symptomatic treatment and aims to achieve the optimal QoL for people within the limits of their diseases.[83] Although rehabilitation practice is based on clinical judgment, and its scientific basis is considered to be weak,[84] scientific evidence is accumulating that rehabilitation is indeed an effective therapeutic intervention.[85]

Despite variations in practice, there is consensus regarding the aims of rehabilitation.[80,81] These are: a comprehensive assessment of physical, psychological and social needs; promotion of physical, psychological and social adaptation to disability and handicap; facilitation of independence in daily activities; maximization of patient and carer satisfaction; empowerment; self-management; and the prevention of complications. The key elements of the rehabilitation process include a multidisciplinary team approach, individually tailored programs and patient-centered function-based goal setting.[86,87]

The World Health Organization's (WHO's) International Classification of Impairments, Disabilities, and Handicaps (ICIDH)[88] is considered to be the cornerstone for evaluating the outcomes of rehabilitation.[89] The ICIDH provides a theory of disablement and the rehabilitation process which has proved to be relevant, easily operationalized and reasonably comprehensive with respect to the aims of rehabilitation. Each of the three concepts can be defined, modified by treatment and measured. Furthermore, as the terminology of the ICIDH is well established, data are universally understood.[89]

At a conceptual level, problems with disability measurement in MS rehabilitation arise from a lack of consensus about definitions, the range of activities to be evaluated and the operational criteria used. Whilst many definitions of disability have been proposed[90–92] and there is agreement that disability refers to disease-related restrictions in activity,[93] there is no agreement concerning the situations in which these restrictions occur. Some authors[94] define disability as ability without reference to situational requirements (e.g. basic abilities such as reaching, bending and dexterity). Others[95] use the term 'functional limitations' to describe such restrictions, and define disability as restrictions in relation to specific domains of a person's own environment, (e.g. personal care and domestic activities). Some authors[96,97] extend the definition of disability to include limitations in performance of socially defined roles and tasks within a sociocultural and physical environment.

These disagreements concerning the basic definition of disability have led to an overlap with other health constructs. Although the WHO attempted to separate disability from impairment and handicap,[98,99] these efforts have only been partially successful.[100,101] Some authors argue that assessing limitations in simple activities measures both impairment and disability,[102] whilst assessing limitations in complex activities measures both disability and handicap.[103,104] The activities to be evaluated by disability measures are also an area of controversy. There are an unlimited number of activities and a wide variety of domains that can be included in disability measures. However, there is no agreement about either.[46,105]

In the field of health outcome measurement, although there is a lack of conceptual clarity regarding these terms, there is broad agreement on the core minimum set of health concepts that should be measured.[106] These include physical health, mental health, social functioning, role functioning and general health perceptions. In MS rehabilitation, these should also include disease-specific (e.g. symptoms), sequelae (e.g. fatigue) and treatment outcomes (e.g. patient/carer satisfaction; self-efficacy, self-management, complications).

Clinician-rated scales

The mainstay of health measurement in MS has been the Kurtzke EDSS,[86] which has superseded the earlier Disability Status Scale.[107] This is an observer (clinician)-rated scale which grades 'disability' due to MS on a continuum of 0 (normal neurological examination) to 10 (death due to MS) in 20 steps. Although the EDSS has been the most widely used measure of outcome in clinical trials of MS,[18,19,108] it has been repeatedly criticized for its poor psychometric properties (i.e. reliability[109,110] and responsiveness[111,112]). The EDSS has not been subjected to comprehensive psychometric evaluation. A distinct advantage of the EDSS is its familiarity as a common language amongst MS rehabilitation clinicians. Unfortunately, this does not guarantee rigorous outcome measurement and, given its scientific properties, this could be considered a lame excuse for the continued usage of the EDSS as the primary outcome measure in treatment trials in MS.

In addition, there are a number of other observer (clinician)-rated scales that measure various aspects of MS symptom manifestation, including the Scripps Neurological Rating Scale,[113] Troiano Functional Scale,[114] European Database for Multiple Sclerosis impairment scale,[115] the Cambridge Multiple Sclerosis Basic Score[116] and the Guys Neurological Disability Scale (GNDS).[117] Although there is variable psychometric evidence to support these, none have been evaluated comprehensively. However, the bigger issue is that clinician-based measures only provide half the picture. Patient-rated scales are required for comprehensive outcome measurement.

In summary, none of the measures above provides the rigorous measurement required to evaluate currently available technologies in MS. All were developed using a common-sense approach based on the intuition and clinical experience of the author rather than in accordance with psychometric principles and item-measurement theory.[118] Patients were rarely directly involved in the construction of these instruments. All are clinician-report (although the GNDS may become self-report) and have the associated problems of observer reliability (inter- and intrarater), limited perspective[119] and methodological limitations for study design.[120]

Patient-rated scales: generic

Although many types of generic measure have been used in MS research, three have been used most frequently: the BI, FIM and Medical Outcomes Study Short Form Health Survey (SF-36).

The BI was developed in 1955 as a simple index of personal activities of daily living.[33,121] Scores for each of its 10 items are summed to give a total score which ranges from 0 (maximum disability) to 20 (minimum disability). The BI is well known to neurologists, has been recommended as a benchmark against which other instruments should be evaluated[84] and has been advocated by the Royal College of Physicians of London as a standard assessment of activities of daily living for elderly persons.[122] A number of studies have addressed its reliability[123–126] and validity[121,127–129] and the available data are very encouraging. Although criticized for its simplicity and lack of responsiveness, this is perhaps surprisingly not confirmed in studies.[130] The major limitation of the BI is that its content is relevant only to people with moderate and severe disability.

The FIM is an 18-item observer-rated instrument which measures disability in terms of burden of care.[131] Each item is rated on a seven-point ordinal scale, and item scores are summed to give six subscales, two domains or a total score. The FIM was specifically developed to fulfill the desperate need for a meaningful outcome measure in medical rehabilitation[34] and, as a consequence, is rapidly becoming the most widely used disability measure. Psychometric data are not extensive but support it as a reliable, valid and responsive measure. The FIM has been used successfully in patients with MS[132,133] but studies of its head-to-head comparison with competing measures (e.g. BI) have yet to be published. Such studies are important as there are financial (US$15 000 per annum) and practical (staff rater requirements) implications associated with its use. Consequently the incremental validity of the FIM above competitors must be demonstrated.

The MOS SF-36 is a 36-item instrument which assesses health status in eight health dimensions by self-reported questionnaire.[35,134] Scores can be derived for each of the eight health dimensions[35] and also two summary scores can be computed.[134]

The reliability and validity of the SF-36 have been the subject of numerous studies which are summarized elsewhere.[35,134] The SF-36 is considered the gold-standard measure of health status and has been referred to as 'a Dow Jones for health' and the optimum outcome measure.[35] Despite these glowing references the SF-36 demonstrates pronounced floor effects and poor responsiveness in patients with advanced disease;[130,135] consequently it is likely to have a limited role in treatment trials of MS. This, in addition to the general limitations generic measures described above, confirms the importance of demonstrating the appropriateness of measurement instruments to the patient populations under study.

Disease-specific scales

There are a number of disease-specific measures available. Of these, three instruments assess general aspects of QoL. The first is the Multiple Sclerosis Quality of Life-54 Instrument (MSQOL-54),[136] which contains 52 items distributed into 12 scales, and two single items. The second is the Functional Assessment Multiple Sclerosis (FAMS),[137] which includes 59 questions, divided into six subscales: mobility, symptoms, emotional well-being (depression), general contentment, thinking/fatigue, and family/social wellbeing. The third is the Leeds Multiple Sclerosis Quality of Life Instrument[138] which includes eight items.

More recently, three disease-specific measures have been developed that propose to tap into specific aspects of MS. The first, the Multiple Sclerosis Impact Scale (MSIS-29), is an instrument measuring the physical (20 items) and psychological (nine items) impact of MS.[139–142] The second, the 12-item MS Walking Scale (MSWS-12), includes 12 items describing the impact of MS on walking. The final measure is the 88-item Multiple Sclerosis Spasticity Scale (MSSS-88) which measures the impact of spasticity in MS.[143]

In summary, these measures provide the potential for rigorous and more targeted measurement required to evaluate MS and its treatment. Each of these measures was developed following psychometric methods, which supports their use in research, but the limitations of disease-specific measures (described above) should also be considered. However, the advent of newer psychometric methodologies may provide new directions for MS rehabilitation measurement such as Rasch item analysis[144] and Item Response Theory (IRT)[145] models.

Conclusions

Increasingly, MS rehabilitation clinicians need to measure unobservable variables. These can be measured rigorously using Likert scales. There are a number of clinician and patient rating scales available for use in MS rehabilitation. When assessing available scales for MS rehabilitation, clinicians must evaluate their clinical usefulness and scientific soundness with respect to a particular study. First, find instruments that can be incorporated into the study design, whose items look like they measure the required constructs for the study (do not be misled by instrument names), and are appropriate to the study sample. Next, examine the empirical evidence that these measures are reliable, valid and responsive in the study sample. Start with evidence for reliability as this is a prerequisite for (but not sufficient for) validity and responsiveness. Next, examine the empirical evidence that the instrument measures what it purports to measure. What type of evidence supports the instrument's validity and how strong is this evidence? Finally, verify that the evidence is there that the instrument has the ability to detect change over time. If no instrument exists and no compromise is acceptable, a new instrument may need to be developed. However, it is important to collaborate with a health measurement expert.

References

1. Ware JE Jr, Brook RH, Davies-Avery A et al. (1980) Conceptualization and Measurement of Health for Adults in the Health Insurance Study: Vol. I, Model of Health and Methodology. Santa Monica, CA, The Rand Corporation.
2. McDowell I, Newell C (1987) Measuring Health: a Guide to Rating Scales and Questionnaires. Oxford, Oxford University Press.
3. Streiner D, Norman GR (1989) Health Measurement Scales: a Practical Guide to Their Development and Use. Oxford, Oxford University Press.
4. Kaska S, Weinstein J (1998) Historical perspective. Ernest Amory Codman, 1869–1940. A pioneer of evidence-based medicine: the end result idea. Spine 23: 629–33.
5. Herndon R (1997) Hand book of neurologic rating scales. New York, Demos Vermande.
6. Visick A (1948) A study of the failures after gastrectomy. Ann R Coll Surg Engl 3: 266.
7. Karnofsky D, Burchenal J (1949) The clinical evaluation of chemotherapeutic agents in cancer. In: Macleod C, ed. Evaluation of

Chemotherapeutic Agents. New York, Columbia University Press: 191–205.

8. Stewart AL, Ware JE Jr, eds (1992) Measuring Functioning and Well-being: the Medical Outcomes Study Approach. Durham, NC, Duke University Press.

9. World Health Organization (1948) Constitution of the World Health Organization. Geneva, WHO Basic Documents.

10. Joralemon D, Fujinaga, K (1997) Studying the quality of life after organ transplantation: research problems and solutions. Soc Sci Med 44: 1259–69.

11. Robinson R (1993) The Policy Context. BMJ 307: 994–6.

12. Streiner DL, Norman GR (1995) Health Measurement Scales: a Practical Guide to Their Development and Use. Oxford, Oxford University Press.

13. Feinstein A (1977) Clinical biostatistics XLI. Hard science, soft data, and the challenge of choosing clinical variables in research. Clin Pharmacol Ther 22: 485–98.

14. Fitzpatrick R, Fletcher A, Gore S et al. (1992) Quality of life measures in health care. I: Applications and issues in assessment. BMJ 305: 1074–7.

15. Fillipi M, Paty DW, Kappos L et al. (1995) Correlations between changes in disability and T2-weighted brain MRI activity in multiple sclerosis: a follow up study. Neurology 45: 255–60.

16. Smith D, Baker GA, Jacoby A, Chadwick DW (1995) The contribution of the measurement of seizure severity to quality of life research. Qual Life Res 4: 143–58.

17. Peto V, Jenkinson C, Fitzpatrick R, Greenhall R (1995) The development and validation of a short measure of functioning and well-being for individuals with Parkinson's disease. Qual Life Res 4: 241–8.

18. IFNB Multiple Sclerosis Study Group (1993) Interferon beta-1b is effective in relapsing–remitting multiple sclerosis. I Clinical results of a multi-centre, randomised, double-blind, placebo-controlled trial. Neurology 43: 655–61.

19. Jacobs LD, Cookfair DL, Rudick RA, Herndon RM (1996) Intramuscular interferon beta-1a for disease progression in relapsing multiple sclerosis. Ann Neurol 39: 285–94.

20. McDonald WI (1995) New treatments for multiple sclerosis. BMJ 310: 345–6.

21. Cleary P, Greenfield S, McNeil B (1991) Assessing quality of life after surgery. Controlled Clin Trials 12: 189s-203s.

22. Bergner M, Rothman M (1987) Health status measures: an overview and guide for selection. Ann Rev Publ Health 8: 191–210.

23. Parkerson G Jr, Broadhead W, Tse C (1995) Health status and severity of illness as predictors of outcomes in primary care. Med Care 33: 53–66.

24. Miilunpalo S, Vuori I, Oja P, Pasanen M, Urponen H (1997) Self-rated health status as a health measure: the predictive value of self-reported health status on the use of physician services and on mortality in the working-age population. J Clin Epidemiol 50: 517–28.

25. Lohr K (1992) Applications of health status assessment measures in clinical practice. Overview of the third conference on advances in health status assessment. Med Care 30: MS1–14.

26. Thurstone LL (1925) A method for scaling psychological and educational tests. J Educ Psychol 16: 433–51.

27. Guttman L (1945) A basis for analysing test–retest reliability. Psychometrika 10: 255–82.

28. Gulliksen H (1950) Theory of Mental Tests. New York, Wiley.

29. Edwards AL (1957) Techniques of Attitude Scale Construction. New York, Appleton-Century-Crofts.

30. Torgerson WS (1958) Theory and Methods of Scaling. New York, John Wiley and Sons.

31. Likert RA (1932) A technique for the development of attitudes. Arch Psychol 140: 5–55.

32. Likert RA, Roslow S, Murphy G (1934) A simple and reliable method of scoring the Thurstone attitude scales. J Social Psychol 5: 228–38.

33. Mahoney FI, Barthel DW (1965) Functional evaluation: the Barthel Index. Md State Med J 14: 61–5.

34. Granger CV, Hamilton BB, Keith RA, Zielezny M, Sherwin FS (1986a) Advances in functional assessment for medical rehabilitation. Topics Geriatr Rehabil 1: 59–74.

35. Ware JE Jr, Snow KK et al. (1993) SF-36 Health Survey Manual and Interpretation Guide. Boston, MA, Nimrod Press.

36. Goldberg DP (1978) Manual of the General Health Questionnaire. Windsor, NFER-Nelson.

37. Zigmond AS, Snaith RP (1983) The Hospital Anxiety and Depression Scale. Acta Psychiatr Scand 67: 361–70.

38. Bowling A (1997) Research Methods in Health: Investigating Health and Health Services. Buckingham, Open University Press.

39. Browne J, McGee H, O'Boyle C (1997) Conceptual approaches to the assessment of quality of life. Psychol Health 12: 737–51.

40. Patrick D, Deyo R (1989) Generic and disease-specific measures in assessing health status and quality of life. Med Care 27: S217–32.

41. Fletcher A, Gore S, Jones D et al. (1992) Quality of life measures in health care. II: Design, analysis, and interpretation. BMJ 305: 1145–8.

42. Dawson J, Fitzpatrick R, Carr A (1996) Questionnaire on the perceptions of patients about total hip replacement. J Bone Joint Surg 78B: 185–90.

43. Fitzpatrick R, Davey C, Buxton M, Jones D (1998) Evaluating

patient-based outcome measures for use in clinical trials. Health Technol Assess 2: i–iv, 1–74.

44. Ruta D, Garratt A, Leng M, Russell I, MacDonald L (1994) A new approach to the measurement of quality of life. The Patient-Generated Index. Med Care 32: 1109–26.

45. Bowling A (1991). Measuring Health: a Review of Quality of Life Measurement Scales. Milton Keynes, Open University Press.

46. Wade DT (1992) Measurement in Neurological Rehabilitation. Oxford, Oxford University Press.

47. McHorney CA, Ware JE Jr, Lu JF, Sherbourne CD (1994) The MOS 36-Item Short-Form Health Survey (SF-36): III. Tests of data quality, scaling assumptions and reliability across diverse patient groups. Med Care 32: 40–66.

48. Ware J, Harris W, Gandek B, Rogers B, Reese P (1997) MAP-R for Windows: Multitrait/Multi-item Analysis Program – Revised Users's Guide Version 1. Boston, MA, Health Assessment Lab.

49. Lohr KN, Aaronson NK, Alonso J et al. (1996) Evaluating quality of life and health status instruments: development of scientific review criteria. Clin Ther 18: 979–92.

50. McHorney CA, Tarlov AR (1995) Individual-patient monitoring in clinical practice: are available health status surveys adequate? Qual Life Res 4: 293–307.

51. Hays R, Anderson R, Revicki D (1993) Psychometric considerations in evaluating health-related quality of life measures. Qual Life Res 2: 441–9.

52. Cronbach L (1951) Coefficient alpha and the internal structure of tests. Psychometrika 16: 297–334.

53. Deyo R, Diehr P, Patrick D (1991) Reproducibility and responsiveness of health status measures. Statistics and strategies for evaluation. Control Clin Trials 12: 142s–58s.

54. Nunnally JC, Bernstein IH (1994) Psychometric Theory. New York, McGraw-Hill.

55. Messick S (1995) Validation of inferences from persons' responses and performances as scientific enquiry into score meaning. Am Psychol 50: 741–49.

56. Kaplan R, Bush J, Berry C (2000) Health status: types of validity and the Index of Well-Being. Health Services Res 478–507.

57. Anastasi A (1986) Evolving concepts of test validation. Ann Rev Psychol 37: 1–15.

58. Cronbach L (1980) Validity on parole: how can we go straight? New Dir Test Meas 5: 99–108.

59. Campbell D, Fiske D (1959) Convergent and discriminant validation by the multi trait-multimethod matrix. Psychol Bull 56: 81–105.

60. Messick S (1980) Test validation and the ethics of assessment. Am Psychol 35: 1012–27.

61. Husted J, Cook R, Farewell V, Gladman D (2000) Methods for assessing responsiveness: a critical review and recommendations. J Clin Epidemiol 53: 459–68.

62. Kazis L, Anderson J, Meenan R (1989) Effect sizes for interpreting changes in health status. Med Care 27: S178–89.

63. Guyatt G, Townsend M, Berman L, Keller J (1987) A comparison of Likert and visual analogue scales for measuring change in function. J Chron Dis 40: 1129–33.

64. Fleiss JL (1986) The Design and Analysis of Clinical Experiments. New York, Wiley.

65. Cone JD, Foster SL (1991) Training in measurement: always the bridesmaid. Am Psychol 46: 653–4.

66. Kurtzke JF (1983) Rating neurological impairment in multiple sclerosis: an expanded disability status scale (EDSS). Neurology 33: 1444–52.

67. Sharrack B, Hughes RAC, Soudain S, Dunn G (1999) The psychometric properties of clinical rating scales used in multiple sclerosis. Brain 122: 141–59.

68. Hobart JC, Freeman JA, Thompson A et al. (2000) Kurtzke scales revisited: the application of psychometric methods to clinical intuition. Brain 123: 1027–40.

69. European Study Group on Interferon beta-1b in Secondary Progressive MS (1998) Placebo-controlled multicentre randomised trial of interferon beta-1b in treatment of secondary progressive multiple sclerosis. Lancet 352: 1491–7.

70. National Institute for Clinical Excellence (2004) Multiple Sclerosis. National Clinical Guideline for Diagnosis and Management in Primary and Secondary Care. London, Royal College of Physicians, 197.

71. Miller DH, Albert PS, Barkhof F et al. (1996) Guidelines for the use of magnetic resonance techniques in monitoring the treatment of multiple sclerosis. Ann Neurol 39: 6–16.

72. Polman CH, Hartung HP (1995) The treatment of multiple sclerosis: current and future. Curr Opin Neurol 8: 200–9.

73. Herndon RM, Murray TJ (1983) Proceedings of the international conference on therapeutic trials in multiple sclerosis. Arch Neurol 40: 663–710.

74. Ellison GW, Myers LW, Leake BD et al. (1994) Design strategies for multiple sclerosis clinical trials. Ann Neurol 36: S108–12.

75. Nauta JJP, Thompson AJ, Barkhof F, Miller DH (1994) Magnetic resonance imaging in monitoring the treatment of multiple sclerosis patients: statistical power of parallel-groups and crossover designs. J Neurol Sci 122: 6–14.

76. Foa R (1996) Ethical considerations raised by clinical trials. In: Goodkin DE, Rudick RA, eds. Multiple sclerosis: advances in clini-

cal trial design, treatment and future perspectives. London, Springer-Verlag: 335–50.

77. Weinshenker BG (1994) Natural history of multiple sclerosis. Ann Neurol 36: S6–S11.

78. Weinshenker BG, Issa M, Baskerville J (1996) Meta-analysis of the placebo-treated groups in clinical trials of progressive MS. Neurology 46: 1613–19.

79. Greenwood RJ, Barnes M, McLellan DL, eds (1993) Neurological Rehabilitation. Edinburgh, Churchill Livingstone.

80. Scheinberg LC (1994) Therapeutic strategies. Ann Neurol 36: S122–9.

81. Thompson AJ (1996) Rehabilitation of progressive neurological disorders: a worthwhile challenge? Opin Neurol 9: 437–40.

82. La Rocca NG, Shapiro RT, Scheinberg LC, Kraft GH (1994) Comprehensive care in multiple sclerosis: the whole versus the parts. J Neurol Rehabil 8: 95–8.

83. McGrath JR, Davis AM (1992) Rehabilitation: where do we go and how do we get there? Clin Rehabil 6: 225–35.

84. Wade DT (1993) Measurement in neurological rehabilitation. Curr Opin Neurol 6: 778–84.

85. Langhorne P, Dennis M, eds (1998) Stroke Units: an Evidence Based Approach. London, British Medical Journal Books.

86. Greenwood RJ (1992) Neurology and rehabilitation in the UK: a view. J Neurol Neurosurg Psychiatry 55: 51–3.

87. Edwards SM (1996) Longer-term management for patients with residual or progressive disability. In: Edwards SM, ed. Neurological Physiotherapy: a Problem-solving Approach. London, Churchill Livingstone: 189–206.

88. World Health Organization (1980) International Classification of Impairments, Disabilities and Handicaps (ICIDH): a manual of classification relating to the consequences of disease. Geneva, World Health Organization.

89. Chamie M (1990) The status and use of the International Classification of Impairments, Disabilities, and Handicaps (ICIDH). World Health Stat Q 43: 273–80.

90. Slater SB, Vukmanovic C, Macukanovic P, Prulovic T, Cutler JL (1974) The definition and measurement of disability. Soc Sci Med 8: 305–8.

91. Krauze EA (1976) The political sociology of rehabilitation. In: Albrecht GL, ed. The Sociology of Physical Disability and Rehabilitation. Pittsburgh, University of Pittsburgh Press.

92. Duckworth D (1983) The Classification and Measurement of Disablement. London, Department of Health and Social Security, Social Research Branch, Research report no. 10.

93. Wood PHN, Badley EM (1981) People with Disabilities. New York, World Rehabilitation Fund.

94. Martin J, Meltzer M, Elliot D (1988) OPCS surveys of disability in Great Britain. Report 1: the Prevalence of Disability Among Adults. London, Her Majesty's Stationery Office.

95. Kempen GIJM, Meedema I, Ormel J, Molenaar W (1996) The assessment of disability with the Groningen Activity Restriction Scale: conceptual framework and psychometric properties. Soc Sci Med 43: 1601–10.

96. Nagi SZ (1979) The concept and measurement of disability. In: Berkowitz ED, ed. Disability policies and government programs. New York, Preager Press: 1–15.

97. Nagi SZ (1991) Disability concepts revisited: implications for prevention. In: Pope AM, Tarlov AR, eds. Disability in America: Toward a National Standard for Prevention. Washington, DC, National Academy Press: 309–39.

98. Badley EM (1987) The ICIDH: format, application in different settings, and distinction between disability and handicap. Int Disabil Stud 9: 122–5.

99. Bury MR (1987) The ICIDH: a review of research and prospects. Int Disabil Stud 9: 118–28.

100. American Medical Association (1984) Guide to the Evaluation of Permanent Impairment, 2nd edn. Chicago, American Medical Association.

101. Mooney V (1987) Impairment, disability, and handicap. Clin Orthop 221: 14–25.

102. Luck JV, Florence DW (1988) A brief history and comparative analysis of disability systems and impairment rating guides. Orthop Clin N Am 19: 839–44.

103. McDowell I, Jenkinson C (1996) Development standards for health measures. J Health Serv Res Policy 1: 238–46.

104. Brook RH, Ware JE Jr, Davies-Avery A et al. (1997) Overview of adult health status measures fielded in RAND's Health Insurance Study. Med care 17(Suppl): 1–131.

105. Keith RA (1984) Functional assessment measures in medical rehabilitation: current status. Arch Phys Med Rehab 65: 74–8.

106. Hunt S (1997) The problem of quality of life. Qual Life Res 6: 205–12.

107. Kurtzke JF (1955) A new scale for evaluating disability in multiple sclerosis. Neurology 5: 580–3.

108. Goodkin DE, Cookfair D, Wende K et al. (1992) Inter- and intra-rater scoring agreement using grades 1.0 to 3.5 of the Kurtzke Expanded Disability Status Scale (EDSS). Neurology 42: 859–63.

109. Willoughby EW, Paty DW (1988) Scales for rating impairment in multiple sclerosis: a critique. Neurology 38: 1793–8.

110. Noseworthy JH, Vander voort MK, Wong CJ, Ebers GC (1990) Interrater variability with the Expanded Disability Status Scale (EDSS)

and Functional Systems (FS) in a multiple sclerosis clinical trial. Neurology 40: 971–5.

111. Whitaker JN, McFarland HF, Rudge P, Reingold SC (1995) Outcomes assessment in multiple sclerosis trials: a critical analysis. Mult Scler 1: 37–47.

112. Hobart JC, Lamping DL, Freeman JA et al. (1997b) Reliability, validity, and responsiveness of the Kurtzke Expanded Disability Status Scale (EDSS) in multiple sclerosis. J Neurol Neurosurg Psychiatry 62: 212

113. Sipe JC, Knobler RL, Braheny SL et al. (1984) A neurological rating scale (NRS) for multiple sclerosis. Neurology 34: 1368–72

114. Cook S, Devereux C, Troiano R et al. (1986) Effect of total lymphoid irradiation in chronic progressive multiple sclerosis. Lancet 1: 1405–9.

115. Confavreux C, Compston DAS, Hommes OR et al. (1992) EDMUS, a European database from multiple sclerosis. J Neurol Neurosurg Psychiatry 55: 671–6.

116. Mumford CJ, Compston A (1993) Problems with rating scales for multiple sclerosis: a novel approach – the CAMBS score. J Neurol 240: 209–15.

117. Sharrack B, Hughes RAC, Soudain S (1996) Guy's Neurological Disability Scale. J Neurol 243(6 Suppl 2): S32.

118. Lord FM (1980) Applications of Item Response Theory to Practical Testing Problems, Hillside, NJ, Lawrence Erlbaum Associates.

119. Sprangers MAG, Aaronson NK (1992) The role of health care providers and significant others in evaluating the quality of life of patients with chronic disease: a review. J Clin Epidemiol 45: 743–60.

120. Hobart JC, Thompson AJ (1996b) Clinical trials of multiple sclerosis. In: Reder AT, ed. Interferon Therapy of Multiple Sclerosis. New York, Marcel Dekker: 4899–508

121. Wylie CM, White BK (1964) A measure of disability. Arch Environ Health 8: 834–9.

122. Royal College of Physicians (1992) Standardised assessment scales for elderly people: report of joint workshops of the Research Unit of the Royal College of Physicians and the British Geriatrics Society. London, Royal College of Physicians of London.

123. Granger CV, Albrecht GL, Hamilton BB (1979) Outcome of comprehensive medical rehabilitation: measurement by PULSES Profile and Barthel Index. Arch Phys Med Rehabil 60: 145–54.

124. Roy CW, Togneri J, Hay E, Pentland B (1988) An inter-rater reliability study of the Barthel Index. Int J Rehabil Res 11: 67–70.

125. Wolfe CDA, Taub NA, Woodrow EJ, Burney PGJ (1991) Assessment of scales of disability and handicap for stroke patients. Stroke 22: 1242–4.

126. Gompertz P, Pound P, Ebrahim S (1993) The reliability of stroke outcome measures. Clin Rehabil 7: 290–6.

127. Wade DT, Langton Hewer R (1987) Functional abilities after stroke: measurement, natural history and prognosis. J Neurol Neurosurg Psychiatry 50: 177–82.

128. McPherson K, Sloan RL, Hunter J, Dowell CM (1993) Validation studies of the OPCS scale – more useful than the Barthel Index? Clin Rehabil 7: 105–12.

129. Gompertz P, Pound P, Ebrahim S (1994) Validity of the extended activities of daily living scale. Clin Rehabil 8: 275–80.

130. Hobart JC, Lamping DL, Freeman JA et al. (1997a) The responsiveness of disability measures in multiple sclerosis. J Neurol Neurosurg Psychiatry 62: 213–14.

131. Hamilton BB, Granger CV, Sherwin FS, Zielezny M, Tashman JS (1987) A uniform national data system for medical rehabilitation. In: Fuhrer MJ, ed. Rehabilitation Outcomes: Analysis and Measurement. Baltimore, MD, Paul H Brookes: 137–47.

132. Brosseau L (1994) The inter-rater reliability and construct validity of the Functional Independence Measure for multiple sclerosis subjects. Clin Rehabil 8: 107–15.

133. Hobart JC, Lamping DL, Freeman JA et al. (1996a) Measuring disability in multiple sclerosis: reliability of the Functional Independence Measure. J Neurol 243 (6 Suppl 2): S32

134. Ware JE Jr, Kosinski MA, Keller SD (1994) SF-36 Physical and Mental Health Summary Scales: a User's Manual. Boston, MA, The Health Institute, New England Medical Centre.

135. Freeman J, Langdon D, Hobart J et al. (1996) The health-related quality of life of people with advanced multiple sclerosis. J Neurol Rehabil 10: 185–94.

136. Vickrey BG, Hays RD, Harooni R et al. (1995) A health-related quality of life measure for multiple sclerosis. Qual Life Res 4: 187–206.

137. Cella DF, Dineen K, Anason B et al. (1996) Validation of the functional assessment of multiple sclerosis quality of life instrument. Neurology 47: 129–39.

138. Ford HL, Tennant A, Johnson MH (1997) The Leeds MSQoL scale: a disease specific measure of quality of life in multiple sclerosis. J Neurol Neurosurg Psychiatry 62(2): 210.

139. Hobart JC, Lamping DL, Fitzpatrick R, Riazi A, Thompson AJ (2001) The Multiple Sclerosis Impact Scale (MSIS-29): a new patient-based outcome measure. Brain 124: 962–73

140. Hobart JC, Riazi A, Lamping DL, Fitzpatrick R, Thompson AJ (2004) Improving the evaluation of therapeutic interventions in multiple sclerosis: development of a patient-based outcome measure. Health Technol Assess 8: 1–60.

141. Hobart JC, Riazi A, Lamping DL, Fitzpatrick R, Thompson AJ (2005) How responsive is the Multiple Sclerosis Impact Scale (MSIS-29)? A comparison with other self-report scales. J Neurol Neurosurg Psychiatry 76: 1539–43

142. Riazi A, Hobart JC, Lamping DL, Fitzpatrick R, Thompson AJ (2002) Multiple sclerosis impact scale (MSIS-29): reliability and validity in hospital-based samples. J Neurol Neurosurg Psychiatry 73: 701–4.

143. Hobart JC, Riazi A, Thompson AJ et al. (2006) Getting the measure of spasticity in MS: the MS Spasticity Scale (MSSS-89). 129: 224–34.

144. Rasch G (1960) Probabilistic Models for Some Intelligence and Attainment Tests. Chicago, University of Chicago Press.

145. Lord FM, Novick MR (1968) Statistical Theories of Mental Test Scores. Reading, MA, Addison-Wesley.

6

Service delivery and models of care in multiple sclerosis

Jennifer A Freeman

Introduction

In recent years there has been an increased awareness of the need for effective healthcare management of people with chronic conditions such as multiple sclerosis (MS), who are major users of long-term care and support services.[1] In part this is because of the recognition of the economic challenge that these conditions pose to the health and social services of all Western countries.[2] As a consequence greater emphasis is now being placed on the importance of paying attention to the method of delivery of services, with some evidence suggesting that the effective organization and delivery of care may have more of an impact on the outcomes of health than investments in medication and technology.[3]

Service delivery encompasses the clinical aspects of what patients and carers need, as well as the organizational, political and financial frameworks of how services are delivered.[4] This chapter will focus predominately on the clinical and organizational aspects of rehabilitation service delivery in MS. It will discuss key concepts underpinning the approach to delivering rehabilitation services, describe current models of care for people with MS, and highlight some of the problems faced when organizing the delivery of these services in an integrated manner.

Approaches to rehabilitation in multiple sclerosis

The multiplicity of symptoms that may arise as a result of MS means that the physical, cognitive and psychosocial consequences of this disease are often wide-ranging, variable and complex. They may evolve over several decades, and last a lifetime. The needs of the person with MS are therefore many and ever changing, extending from the core medical parameters to include every facet of individual, family and community existence.[5] As a consequence it is now widely acknowledged that effective rehabilitation strategies, involving the knowledge, expertise and collaboration of a wide range of different health and social care professionals, are paramount to the overall management of people with MS.[6,7] Effective management is characterized by a multidisciplinary team approach with professionals working across organizational boundaries, using evidence-based treatment plans to provide care based on the individual needs of the patient, and with a key worker to co-ordinate care.[6]

To generalize, the provision of rehabilitation for people with MS can broadly be described as falling into three main categories:

- Education and health promotion
- Restorative rehabilitation
- Maintenance rehabilitation

When viewed together they can be seen as providing a continuum of rehabilitation care in which a different emphasis is placed on different aspects of the rehabilitation process throughout different stages of the disease process. They are briefly summarized as follows.

Education and health promotion

The pursuit of personal health and wellness is as important to those with chronic disease as it is to the general population and, as such, it is recognized that health promotion is an underlying goal that should drive all aspects of rehabilitation.[8] In response to this, there is now a greater emphasis on ensuring that education about living with the condition, and maintaining a healthy lifestyle is incorporated as a routine part of healthcare delivery in the early stages of the disease. This requires an active process of education and self-management wherein the person with MS begins to recognize problems (and potential problems) as they arise, and learns how to adapt to and manage some of the challenges that confront them. A variety of different interventions are used to help achieve this, which include: educational courses, self-management programs such as the Expert Patient program,[9] and exercise and fitness groups.[10] In line with the view that wellness encompasses physical, emotional, occupational, social and intellectual factors, there has also been an increased emphasis on forging links with services outside the healthcare arena, such as local leisure centers, the workplace and voluntary organizations.

Restorative rehabilitation

In general people are referred for rehabilitation after they have lost an important function or are experiencing difficulty maintaining their usual roles, due either to acute changes following a relapse, or to deterioration as a consequence of disease progression. Restorative rehabilitation focuses on maximizing quality of life by restoring lost abilities so as to enable the person to function at their optimal capacity within the limits of their disease. Typically this type of rehabilitation is provided when the level of disability is mild to moderate. The rehabilitation episode is time limited, relatively short in duration, and is aimed at achieving specific measurable goals, with success often being measured in fairly concrete terms of improvements in functional ability.[11] It can be provided within an inpatient setting (either acute hospital or a rehabilitation unit),[12–14] as an outpatient,[15] or within the community.[16] Improvements can be achieved through a variety of different interventions which include those aimed at:

- Directly improving existing physical, emotional and cognitive impairments, such as improving strength and range of motion; reducing hypertonicity, reducing depression, and improving bladder and bowel control.
- Involving processes that are clearly distinct from biological recovery, and include learning, the acquisition of new skills and the changing of behavior.[17] These strategies tend to be used when impairments cannot be reversed.

Unlike in acute and reversible illnesses, rehabilitation in MS is never 'one off'.[18] Indeed a key aim of rehabilitation in MS is to help the person adjust to and cope with the varying disabling consequences of the disease, by adapting and readapting to MS repeatedly over time.[19] It is therefore often appropriate that, during the course of the disease, restorative rehabilitation be undertaken on a repeated basis, and across the variety of different settings. The key factor for determining whether and when further rehabilitation is required is that clearly identifiable goals can be set that can be achieved over a time-limited period.[11]

Maintenance rehabilitation

The high costs of secondary complications, which include contractures, pressure sores, depression, disuse weakness, unemployment and carer ill-health have been widely acknowledged, both in economic and quality of life terms.[7] The key aim of maintenance rehabilitation is to maintain function within the limits of the progression of the disease by, wherever possible, preventing these avoidable and unwanted secondary complications from developing, or arresting or improving them once they have occurred.[18]

As is characteristic of any rehabilitation approach, a multidisciplinary team is involved in providing a wide range of interventions, which can be focused at different levels, including:

*   Impairments, by focusing on aspects such as the implementation of regimens to maintain or improve range of motion, strength, pressure care and postural alignment; or by providing counseling and emotional support where necessary
*   Function, for example by maintaining independence through the use of aids and equipment, or by ensuring that adequate personal help is provided
*   Preservation of safety, for example in functions such as transfers

Unfortunately people with MS are most often referred for maintenance rehabilitation in the later stages of the disease, when disability is severe and when secondary complications have already begun to develop or, as too often is the case, have become well established. This can also be a time when cognitive difficulties may make it difficult for the person to effectively manage their own care. As a consequence staff members are often faced with a complex web of interrelated impairments and functional deficits which can be extremely difficult and time consuming to manage. A further challenge to effective management is that maintenance rehabilitation is commonly provided within the community, either in the patient's own home or in long-term institutional care. In these environments organization of care and communication between staff is often complicated by the fact that the teams involved are usually large in number and include qualified and unqualified staff from both healthcare and social service organizations. Ensuring that input from such a diverse range of people across different organizations occurs appropriately and to a high standard is fraught with difficulties, and raises numerous challenges, which include determining how best to organize ongoing training, to ensure clear communication with regard to changes in circumstances and routines, and to establish common protocols for care. The case management approach is one way of attempting to tackle these difficulties particularly in people with more complex and long-term needs.[20]

Although considered a high priority by people with MS and their carers, funding for the provision of services designed to deliver maintenance rehabilitation over the longer term has proven universally difficult to attain, not only in MS, but across the broad range of disabling neurological diseases.[6,7] This is not helped by the fact that little evidence exists to demonstrate its benefit. As a consequence the burden of long-term care and maintenance therapy often falls on the carer, and carer burnout and emotional distress is common.[21,22] This burden can be lessened by active and sustained follow-up wherein the patient's health status is monitored, potential complications are identified, and progress is checked and reinforced on implementation of the care plan.[23] This can be achieved in a variety of different ways including: the provision of self-referral systems which allow individuals the flexibility to access services when their needs change; scheduled return visits at regular intervals, such as those commonly provided by outpatient medical reviews; or by telephone contact services.

It is clearly simplistic to describe rehabilitation as neatly falling into these three distinct categories. In reality it tends to be amalgamated into one rather amorphous approach, where rehabilitation and care are intertwined. Nevertheless it provides a relatively simple framework for describing the key aims of different services, and may be helpful in trying to understand the reasoning behind the development of different models of care in MS.

Current models of rehabilitation care in multiple sclerosis

It is not unreasonable to expect that clinical needs be central in informing and shaping the development of services and that, as a consequence, there might exist a universally acceptable model of rehabilitation care for people with MS. In practice, historical patterns of service delivery and resource issues (which are heavily influenced by the political decision-making process) are key drivers in the process of service development.[4] As a consequence there is no agreed model for the organization of MS rehabilitation services, with care being delivered in many different ways, varying from society to society and culture to culture.[24]

The structure and funding mechanism of the healthcare system appears to have perhaps the greatest influence on the model of care provided in each country. For example, in some countries patients are routinely offered inpatient treatment on an annual basis[25] whereas in others patients are selectively admitted according to current needs.[12] Differences in the availability of specialist MS facilities (inpatient and outpatient) are also apparent. These were highlighted in a survey undertaken by the International Federation of Multiple Sclerosis Societies.[26] Of the 26 countries surveyed, 25 countries offered general consultation services, but only 16 provided speciality outpatient care, and 11 specialist inpatient care. These inequalities exist, not only between nations, but also within nations. For example, in the UK it is now widely acknowledged that regional variations exist in both the range of services available and the ease of accessibility to these services, resulting in widespread inequality of care provision.[6]

Promoting specialist rehabilitation care

Rehabilitation can be provided within a specialist or a generalist environment. There is ongoing discussion and debate as to which approach best serves the needs of people with MS. Although the evidence to support one approach over another within the field of MS is scant, surveys of people with MS highlight that their preference is for specialist services;[27] and there is strong evidence from other long-term neurological conditions such as stroke[28] that specialist rehabilitation services achieve better outcomes compared with generalist care, and are more highly valued by patients. This has also been found to be the case for a range of other long-term non-neurological conditions, such as cancer.[29]

In contrast to more common conditions such as stroke and cancer, the incidence and prevalence of MS means that many health services lack the necessary critical mass of patients to justify the development of a condition-specific service. As a consequence a specialist neurorehabilitation (as distinct from an MS-specific) approach to the rehabilitation management of people with MS is strongly supported by current guidelines and expert consensus documents across a range of countries.[6,19,30,31] The thrust of the argument supporting this approach is that specialized services reorganize care in a more efficient and effective manner by bringing together the personnel and resources required to meet the needs of the patient. This seems to be particularly beneficial when needs are complex, and where health professionals need to be seeing enough patients to understand the complex issues and to develop and maintain the necessary skill level. Importantly there is some evidence to suggest that patients are also more satisfied[32,33] and confident[34] with the care they receive from specialist services.

In reality, practical factors, such as the availability of specialist staff and facilities, means that there is currently a mixed approach to rehabilitation of people with MS in the UK. The bulk of rehabilitation is delivered by generic rehabilitation or general neurological services (across hospital, inpatient rehabilitation and community settings), and is complemented by regional specialist neurorehabilitation services. These regional services include: specialist inpatient neurorehabilitation units; specialist outpatient services based around the management of complex symptoms (such as spasticity, continence and pain); complex interventions (such as seating and posture and functional electrical stimulation); or specialist community rehabilitation teams.[35] Unlike stroke rehabilitation, where stroke units are considered the gold standard of care,[28] it is rare in the UK for services to be MS-specific, although this is a more common model of rehabilitation care in some European countries.[25,36]

Towards a collaborative 'whole systems' approach to care delivery

It is clear that a single setting or service cannot adequately meet a person's needs across the lifelong course of MS. As a consequence individuals need to access different services, for different reasons, at different points in time.

An inevitable consequence of this is that people need to be transferred between services and organizations. This often results in fragmentation of the delivery of care, and it is not uncommon for confusion and anxiety to arise in patients, carers and professionals alike. While these problems are common to the management of all neurological disorders, they are often magnified in MS due to the unpredictability, variability and lifelong nature of the condition. Managing this complexity in practice is extremely difficult, and unfortunately there are no easy solutions to these problems 'since it requires a multiplicity of agencies, professions and services to work together, even though they are all funded, managed and held accountable though different means'.[37]

Pathways of care

In an attempt to address this fragmentation of care delivery, efforts are now being made in the UK to develop a coherent 'whole systems' approach to the delivery of rehabilitation care, wherein collaborative working extends across the full spectrum of rehabilitation services. The rationale underlying this approach is that the unique needs of individuals can be satisfactorily met only by enabling the person to follow different 'pathways of care' throughout the whole system. In this approach it is advocated that all parts of the healthcare system, social services and other statutory services have joint responsibility for rehabilitation care, and should work collaboratively using agreed protocols, to ensure that the different services are working towards achieving a common 'patient-centered' goal.[6] Table 6.1 provides a schema of this system of care delivery.

The delivery of potential pathways of care is clearly dependent upon the availability and accessability of relevant services, and the appropriate and timely referral of persons to these services. There is evidence to suggest, however, that referral to required services are often not based upon clinical need, but rather are heavily influenced by factors such as socioeconomic status, levels

Table 6.1. Rehabilitation services for people with MS. A collaborative 'whole systems' approach to care delivery

Hospital	Intensive rehabilitation	Intermediate services	Community-based services
Diagnostic clinics	Specialist inpatient rehabilitation units	Community hospitals	Community rehabilitation within the person's home setting
Multidisciplinary clinics, e.g. – assessment clinics – relapse clinics – spasticity clinics – continence services	General inpatient rehabilitation units	Respite care services	Links with specialist vocational services; assessments within the workplace; liaison with local employment services
Inpatient rehabilitation, e.g. during relapse management; with surgical procedures such as intrathecal baclofen pumps			Links with social services providing personal care and support within the person's home
Outpatient rehabilitation			Links with voluntary organizations, e.g. MS Society
			Day hospitals
			Links with local leisure centers

of health, the funding mechanisms within the healthcare system and biases of clinicians working within it.[38] The development of national[6,30] and international[19,31] recommendations for care is an attempt to begin to tackle some of these problems. Once these guidelines and recommendations are established, the use of mechanisms such as integrated care pathways and protocols of care provide a helpful structure for clarifying the processes involved, and evaluating whether they are adhered to.[39]

Determining the optimum pathway of care for an individual

No two people with MS are the same. The goal of care pathways is to make sure that the individual with MS receives the best care, in the best place, from the best person or team. Clinical need is clearly a key consideration when making decisions about where care should be best delivered for the person with MS. It is, however, not the only factor to consider. The physical, cognitive and emotional needs of the individual and their family/carers should also be taken into account. For instance, the personal preferences of the person with MS, and lifestyle issues such as family and work considerations, are key to the decision-making process, but often appear to be neglected in practice.[40] Staff must also consider the psychological impact of the rehabilitation setting and the timing of rehabilitation upon the person and how this might affect their ability or desire to actively participate in the rehabilitation process. Economic and practical considerations will also play a role in determining the chosen care pathway. For instance, the team needs to consider physical factors within the treatment settings that will affect the intervention, such as the staff resources available both in terms of skill level and staff numbers, the amount of space to carry out proposed activities, the equipment available, how much time is available for assessment and management, or how much assistance can be accessed for more complex situations. All of these are important considerations in determining the optimum pathway of care for an individual.

Often a number of options exist with regard to the pathway of care available to the person with MS. During an acute attack, for example, steroid therapy in collaboration with rehabilitation could be provided either within a hospital environment or within the person's own home environment. Where the problems are complex and interrelated, a period of inpatient rehabilitation may be the optimal choice of management, enabling intensive daily multidisciplinary input to achieve improvements. On some occasions, however, an inpatient admission might be far from ideal and perhaps even counterproductive. For instance, when the main aim of intervention is to teach the carer suitable techniques to help care for their severely disabled spouse, rehabilitation within the home environment is likely to be more relevant and effective. In other instances, when the problems experienced are relatively straightforward, outpatient intervention may be effective in addressing problems while having the advantage of enabling home and work life to continue relatively undisturbed. For many people access to all of these services may be necessary at some stage of the disease course. Determining which rehabilitation service and approach best meets the needs of the individual at a specific point in time, requires a comprehensive assessment of needs from someone who has specialist experience and skill as well as local knowledge about the various options that are available. It requires those involved to reflect upon and answer a number of rather simple but searching questions (Box 6.1).

Box 6.1. Questions to ask when evaluating service delivery

Is the person getting the most appropriate care?
Is the most appropriate person giving the care?
Is the care being given at the most appropriate time?
Is the care being given in the ideal place?

Key considerations in the delivery of a collaborative model of rehabilitation care

There are a number of important features in this proposed model of care. These include the following.

Assessment and selection

A detailed, accurate and comprehensive assessment of the needs of the person with MS and their carer is essential to determine the specific areas that rehabilitation may benefit at a single point in time. It has been emphasized throughout this chapter that this assessment process is most effective when undertaken by professionals with specialist knowledge of rehabilitation and MS.[41] Such an assessment enables individual care plans to be formulated and implemented according to individual need and to the patient's personal preference.

Partnership

It is generally accepted that rehabilitation outcomes are enhanced by effective collaboration between the person with a long-term condition, their families and the team of professionals involved in their care.[23] Negotiation and co-operation is required for such partnership to develop and be sustained. This relies upon professionals providing information in clear and simple language that is meaningful and relevant to the person with MS. It requires professionals to use their own expertise, but also to acknowledge the expertise of people with MS, who have often lived with their disability for a long time and who are therefore 'experts' as to their own specific needs.[42] It requires the professional to support the patient's personal experiential knowledge base by providing advice and guidance to help prepare them to manage their health and healthcare by using effective and practical self-management strategies.[43] Rehabilitation strategies such as goal setting, action planning, problem solving and follow-up are available to assist the professional in developing a sustained working relationship with individuals.[44] This partnership must extend beyond the person with MS to include carers and family members, particularly when cognitive and physical difficulties mean that the person becomes reliant on others for aspects such as self-care and making decisions related to their daily life.

Co-ordination of care by a key worker

In both the UK and the USA, specialist MS nurse roles are increasingly advocated in an attempt to minimize some of the problems generated by fragmented care-delivery systems. A key part of the role of MS specialist nurses is that they act as a 'key worker' or co-ordinator of services, to ensure that a holistic, client-centered approach is taken and that continuity of care and communication between services is facilitated.[45] Case manager roles within the community care setting are also beginning to be established for the management of those people with more complex disability,[20] in an attempt to facilitate care which is provided across multiple organizations and across different settings. General practitioners clearly also have a fundamental role to play as co-ordinators and communicators within the system.

Effective communication

There is a responsibility on all members involved in the delivery of rehabilitation to provide timely and informed handover from one team to another to enhance the provision of effective care. This should include documentation which not only provides information on the medical aspects of the condition, but also knowledge (which is usually accumulated in the head) about the patient's preferences, values and context, since this is especially important for bridging separate care events and ensuring that services are responsive to need.[46] Integrated healthcare records which enable information to be shared by all care providers is one practical means of improving communication and continuity of care between services.[44] The development of outreach and in-reach therapy and nursing posts may also go some way to improving communication, as well as beginning to bridge the cultural gap which very often exists between health and social service organizations. Importantly these approaches also facilitate the use of rehabilitation strategies such as goal setting across organizations. It seems reasonable to anticipate that these developments may enhance both the continuity and the patient-centered approach to the care delivered.

Clear and transparent referral mechanisms

Referral mechanisms within and between services need to be clear and transparent to both the person with MS and those professionals working with them. Clear guidance as to who and how someone may benefit from the service is important in facilitating good communication and shared decision-making. While integrated care pathways and protocols of care have been demonstrated to be useful in achieving this within single services,[39] to date they have proven notoriously difficult to implement across settings such as community teams, where there are wider organizational barriers.[47]

Summary and conclusions

Multiple sclerosis challenges health and social care providers throughout the spectrum of the disease. Its variable course, variety of symptoms and wide variety of care needs demands broad-based, dynamic and collaborative models of care involving many professionals in health and allied services.

Currently no universally acceptable model of MS rehabilitation care exists. Whilst the evidence base to support the efficacy of individual rehabilitation services is slowly expanding, it remains relatively limited and is compromised by difficulties in trial design.[48] Care therefore must be taken when interpreting studies and extrapolating data into different settings. Currently inpatient assessment and rehabilitation has the strongest evidence base to support this approach in improving function and quality of life. More studies are starting to emerge supporting community care. There are still several areas, however, where there is a dearth of information about effectiveness. For instance, no studies have described or explored the effectiveness of rehabilitation when it spans different settings and organizations. In part this is due to the difficulties in undertaking scientifically credible and clinically meaningful research within this area. It is important, therefore, not simply to dismiss these different rehabilitation interventions and models of care on the basis of inadequate evidence for efficacy, since the lack of evidence does not equate to evidence for a lack of efficacy. There is clearly an urgent need for further studies to be undertaken to inform the debate.

Questions relating to the best model of care in terms of specific aspects of rehabilitation service delivery such as who should have it, when, where, for what, by whom, in what setting and for how long are extraordinarily difficult and a long way from being solved. Interdisciplinary and interorganizational working within and outside the healthcare arena is almost certainly the way forward. It is suggested that only through effective liaison and collaborative working between these different organizations can the existing fragmented service provision be brought together to provide the much-needed improvements in quality of care that all those affected by MS deserve.

References

1. Hoffman C, Rice D, Sung HY (1996) Persons with chronic conditions: their prevalence and costs. JAMA 276: 1473–9.
2. Holmes J, Madgwick T, Bates D (1995) The cost of multiple sclerosis. Br J Econ 8: 181–93.

3. Epping-Jordan J, Bengoa R, Kawar R, Sabate E (2001) The challenge of chronic conditions: WHO responds. BMJ 323: 941–8.

4. Robertson D (2003) Developing and delivering services for people with Parkinson's disease. In: Playford ED, ed. Queen Square Rehabilitation Series: Rehabilitation of Parkinson's Disease. London, Martin Dunitz: 83–103.

5. Perry S (1994) Living with Multiple Sclerosis. Newcastle upon Tyne, Atheneum Press Ltd.

6. National Institute for Clinical Excellence (2003) Multiple sclerosis: management of multiple sclerosis in primary and secondary care. Clin Guideline 8.

7. Department of Health (2005) National Service Framework for long-term conditions. Available at http://www.dh.gov.uk/assetRoot/04/10/53/69/04105369.pdf. Accessed January 2006

8. Stuifbergen AK, Rogers S (1997) Health promotion: an essential component of rehabilitation for persons with chronic disabling conditions. Adv Nurs Sci 19: 1–20.

9. Department of Health (2001) The Expert Patient: a new approach to chronic disease management for the 21st century. London, Department of Health.

10. Petajan JH, Gappmaier E, White AT et al. (1996) Impact of aerobic training on fitness and quality of life in multiple sclerosis. Ann Neurol 39: 432–41

11. Thompson AJ (2001) Symptomatic management and rehabilitation in multiple sclerosis. J Neurol Neurosurg Psychiatry 71(Suppl 2): ii22–ii27.

12. Freeman JA, Langdon DW, Hobart JC, Thompson AJ (1997) The impact of inpatient rehabilitation on progressive multiple sclerosis. Ann Neurol 42: 236–44.

13. Solari A, Filippini G, Gasco P et al. (1999) Physical rehabilitation has a positive effect on disability in multiple sclerosis patients. Neurology 52: 57–62

14. Craig J, Young CA, Ennis M et al. (2003) A randomised controlled trial comparing rehabilitation against standard therapy in multiple sclerosis patients receiving intravenous steroid treatment. J Neurol Neurosurg Psychiatry 74: 1225–30

15. Patti F, Ciancio MR, Cacopardo M et al. (2003) Effects of a short outpatient rehabilitation treatment on disability of multiple sclerosis patients: a randomised controlled trial. J Neurol 250: 861–6

16. Pozzilli C, Brunetti M, Amicosante AMV et al. (2002) Home based management in multiple sclerosis: results of a randomized controlled trial. J Neurol Neurosurg Psychiatry 73: 250–5

17. McLellan L (2002) The future of rehabilitation: rehabilitation should be regarded as a scientific challenge [Letters]. BMJ 324: 737.

18. Ward CD, Phillips M, Smith A, Moran M (2003) Multidisciplinary approaches in progressive neurological disease: can we do better? J Neurol Neurosurg Psychiatry 74(Suppl 4): iv8–iv12

19. European Multiple Sclerosis Platform (2004) Recommendations on Rehabilitation Services for Persons with Multiple Sclerosis in Europe. Italy, Assocazione Italiana Sclerosis Multipla.

20. Murphy E (2004) Case management and community matrons for long term conditions. BMJ 329: 1251–2

21. Carton H, Loos R, Pacolet J et al. (2000) A quantitative study of unpaid care giving in multiple sclerosis. Mult Scler 6: 274–9.

22. McKeown LP, Porter-Armstrong AP, Baxter GD (2003) The needs and experiences of caregivers of individuals with multiple sclerosis: a systematic review. Clin Rehab 17: 234–8.

23. Von Korff M, Gruman J, Schaefer J et al. (1997) Collaborative management of chronic illness. Ann Intern Med 127: 1097–102.

24. Wade D (1997) Services for patients with multiple sclerosis [Editorial]. J Neurol Neurosurg Psychiatry 63: 275–8.

25. Vaney C (1992) The MS Rehabilitation Centre in Montana, Switzerland – present situation. In: Ketelaer P, Battaglia M, eds. Rehabilitation in Multiple Sclerosis (RIMS): Proceedings of the First European Workshop. Genoa, Italy: Assocazione Italiana Sclerosis Multipla: 101–3.

26. Paty DW (1994) Overall summary of the survey of long term care strategies for patients with multiple sclerosis. MS Manage 1: 22–7.

27. Somerset M, Campbell R, Sharp DJ et al. (2001) What do people with MS want and expect from MS Services? Health Expect 4: 29–37.

28. Stroke Unit Trialists' Collaboration (1997) Collaborative systematic review of the randomized trial of organized inpatient (stroke unit) care after stroke. BMJ 314: 151–9.

29. Selby P, Gillis C, Haward R (1996) Benefits from specialised cancer care. Lancet 348: 313–18.

30. Medical Advisory Board of the National Multiple Sclerosis Society (2004) Rehabilitation: Recommendations for Persons with Multiple Sclerosis Expert Opinion Paper. Available at http://www.nationalmssociety.org/PRC.asp Accessed January 2006.

31. Multiple Sclerosis International Federation (2005) Principles to Promote the Quality of Life in People with Multiple Sclerosis. Available at http://www.msif.org/docs/PrinciplestoPromoteQualityofLife1.pdf. Accessed January 2006.

32. Schwartz CE, Brotman S, LaRocca N, Lee H (1998) Patient perception of quality of care provided by specialists and generalists. Mult Scler 4: 426–32

33. Wade D (2001) A Study of Services for Multiple Sclerosis: Lessons for Managing Chronic Disability. London, Royal College of Physicians.

34. Vickrey BG, Edmonds ZV, Shatin D et al. (1999) General neurologist and subspecialist care for multiple sclerosis: patients' perceptions. Neurology 53: 1190–7.

35. Makepeace RW, Barnes MP, Semlyn JK, Stevenson J (2001) The establishment of a community multiple sclerosis team. Int J Rehabil Res 24: 137–41.

36. Mostert S, Kesselring J (2002) Effects of a short-term training program on aerobic fitness, fatigue, health perception and activity level of subjects with multiple sclerosis. Mult Scler 8: 161–8.

37. Audit Commission (2000) The Way to Go Home: Rehabilitation and Remedial Services for Older People. Northampton, UK, Belmont Press.

38. Beatty PW, Hagglund KJ, Neri MT et al. (2003) Access to health care services among people with chronic or disabling conditions: patterns and predictors. Arch Phys Med Rehabil 84: 1417–25.

39. Rossiter DA, Edmondson A, Al Shahi R, Thompson AJ (1998) Integrated care pathways in multiple sclerosis rehabilitation: completing the audit cycle. Mult Scler 4: 85–9.

40. Robinson I, Hunter M, Neilson S (1996) A Dispatch from the Frontline: the Views of People with Multiple Sclerosis About Their Needs. A Qualitative Approach. London, Brunel MS Research Unit.

41. Johnson J, Thompson AJ (1996) Rehabilitation in a neuroscience centre: the role of expert assessment and selection. Br J Ther Rehabil 3: 303–8.

42. Freeman JA, Edwards MS (1999) Whose life is it anyway? [Editorial]. Physiother Res Int 4: ii-iv.

43. Hatch J (1997) Building partnerships. In: Thompson AJ, Polman C, Hohlfeld R, eds. Multiple Sclerosis: Clinical Challenges and Controversies. London, Martin Dunitz: 345–53.

44. Lewis R, Dixon J (2004) Rethinking management of chronic diseases. BMJ 328: 220–2.

45. Forbes A, While A, Dyson L et al. (2003) Impact of clinical nurse specialists in multiple sclerosis – synthesis of the evidence. J Adv Nurs 42: 442–62.

46. Haggerty JL, Reid RJ, Freeman GK (2003) Continuity of care: a multidisciplinary review. BMJ 327: 1219–21.

47. Rees G, Huby G, McDade L, McKechnie L (2004) Joint working in community mental health teams: implementation of an integrated care pathway. Health Soc Care Commun 12: 527–36.

48. Kesselring J, Beer S (2005) Symptomatic therapy and neuro-rehabilitation in multiple sclerosis. Lancet Neurol 4: 643–52.

Index